PATHWAYS OF TEACHING NURSING: KEEPING IT REAL!

Sylvia Rayfield & Loretta Manning

ICAN PUBLISHING INC.
P.O. Box 6192
Bossier City, Louisiana 71171
1-866-428-5589
www.icanpublishing.com

Cover Design by Diane Kostick, Starnet Media Group, Allendale, New Jersey

ICAN Publishing Inc.
P.O. Box 6192
Bossier City, Louisiana 71171-6192
www.icanpublishing.com

This publisher is dedicated to provide competent and reliable information regarding the subject matter covered. However, it is sold with the understanding that the authors and publisher are not engaged in rendering legal or other professional advice. Nurse Practice Acts often vary from state to state and if legal or other expert assistance is required, the services of a professional should be sought. The authors and publisher specifically disclaim any liability that is incurred from the use or application of the contents of this book.

ISBN# 0-9761029-1-9

Library of Congress Publication Data

Rayfield, Sylvia and Loretta Manning
Pathways of Teaching Nursing: Keeping It Real
First Edition January 2006

TITLES BY SYLVIA RAYFIELD & LORETTA MANNING

NCLEX-RN™ 101: How To Pass
(Now in fifth edition)

NURSING MADE INSANELY EASY
(Now in forth edition)

PHARMACOLOGY MADE INSANELY EASY
(Now in second edition)

PATHWAYS OF TEACHING NURSING: KEEPING IT REAL!

ICAN PUBLISHING INC.

Preface

PATHWAYS OF TEACHING NURSING: KEEPING IT REAL

"We are what we think. All that we are arises with our thoughts.
With our thoughts we make the world."
From "The Dhammapada: Sayings of the Buddha"

This book has been written by Sylvia Rayfield and Loretta Manning. We have been teachers of nursing students and mentors for nursing faculty for over 45 years. Our experience as consultants to all types of nursing education programs has provided us with unique experiences in conferring with Associate, Baccalaureate, and Diploma nursing programs all over the United States and in some international countries.

Students and faculty who have attended our presentations have asked for this book for many years. Students have wanted a way to learn complicated material and remember what they have learned. Nurse educators have requested strategies to teach complicated material in ways that students can remember.

This book is written to inspire nursing faculty to reach a higher plane than is often used in teaching students of nursing. Pathways in this book will transform teachers toward revolutionizing the relationship between faculty and student with an accord that both are learners and that we are in this together. *These are more than the Pathways of Teaching Nursing. They are paths for life.* Trust that the teaching-learning process can be used as a platform to provide tools that learners can utilize at every juncture of their lives.

We dedicate this work to nursing faculty that are striving for PATHWAYS that will provide excellence in their teaching experience.

Sylvia Rayfield
Loretta Manning

Acknowledgements

Jackie McVey, PhD, a published, creative and well known nurse educator agreed to write the introductory chapter. Jackie has been in our lives for many years and made many valuable contributions to our books. She is currently professor of nursing at the University of Texas, Tyler. Dr. McVey has an exceptional way with words and has described our endeavors in a matchless first chapter. We are deeply grateful for her wisdom, enthusiasm, encouragement and acceptance of what some educators are considering unheard of methods. Jackie has used the methods and knows they work.

Darlene Franklin, M.N. has written the technology chapter in this book, because she is our expert on the ins and outs of "high tech". She has been a creative contributor to our books for many years. Darlene has many years of experience in teaching "just about everything in the nursing curriculum" with flair, grace and the savvy that comes from loving the students. Her work in South Africa, Sweden, and many other parts of the world is recognized as valuable contributions to the nursing profession. We are indebted to Darlene for her research and experience with the technology discussed in this chapter. She is currently Assistant Professor at Tennessee Technological University in Cookeville, Tennessee.

Melissa Geist, PhD, added research credibility to this book thru the *Afterword*. Melissa attended one of our workshops where we made the comment that this material had not been published in the nursing literature. She loudly commented that it may not be in nursing literature, but is certainly in the science literature. She agreed to write the last chapter to show the relationship between this research and our experience.

We could not write a contributor page without acknowledging the many nursing faculty that we have worked with over the 25 years that we have been in business. It has been gratifying to see many of them accept the pathways and tell us how much easier their life is, how much more fun they are having and how the students love their new approach.

We are truly appreciative of the support of our families. Their love provides the foundation for our creativity. Thank you Randy, Juanita, Erica, Burger, Tina, Alita and families.

Table of Contents

Preface

Acknowledgements

Chapter 1

PATHWAYS OF TEACHING NURSING: KEEPING IT REAL

Jackie McVey, PhD, RN

Like a compass that guides adventurers through wilderness territory, the "teach the teachers" insights in this book have as their dual purposes to both focus and empower the work of nurse educators. These themes of focus on priorities and empowerment through the teacher-student relationship are repeatedly emphasized in all the chapters.

Nursing is an application profession with high academic and performance standards. The main desire of nurse educators is that all the students they teach will become safe, effective, and successful professional nurses. Our commitment to promoting quality nursing care requires faculty to be "gatekeepers" on behalf of public stakeholders who want our programs to maintain standards of excellence.

Unfortunately, our zeal for excellence sometimes causes us to be unintentional gatekeepers. We can block student learning and skills development by using flawed teaching strategies. Results at times include substandard student performance, low licensure examination scores, poor student and nurse retention rates, low morale, and even bitter attitudes among individuals capable of becoming fine professional nurses. This book addresses these dilemmas with down to earth approaches that are wise, enthusiastic, motivating, and even fun. While the educational preparation of nurses is serious business, who says it has to be boring?

FOCUS

The "focus" aim of teaching nursing has been vividly illustrated in several ways throughout the chapters of this book. The main characteristic of focus for teaching nursing is the provision of "virtual reality" priority setting on content, judgment, and skills. The idea at every point is to "Keep it real" and thus interesting and usable in actual nursing situations. Three areas are integrated into all areas covered in this book. (MAP)

MAP	
M	mastery Concepts for classroom, lab, and clinical assignments
A	achieve reality based clinical experiences
P	participation is active through exercises to engage students and keep them focused on learning

Mastery Concepts:

Mastery concepts are the "takeaway" knowledge, judgments, and skills that we want students to recall, apply, and revise during weeks, months, and years. There are two categories of mastery concepts:

The "What" of Mastery Concepts:

1. Mandatories. Essential topics and skills required by professional licensing and accreditation boards and professional organizations (Boards of Nurse Examiners, ANA, NLN, AACN, NCLEX Review Council, JCAHO and other health agency accrediting boards. Examples: Infection control, emergency responses, health promotion.

2. Main unique points of each type content and skills. Clusters of concepts related to the topic to be learned. Includes accumulated knowledge on what is currently known and what works in clinical settings. Best if limited in number, since we have better recall when a topic is reduced to a few main concepts that capture the essence of its characteristics and significance.

The "So What" of Mastery Concepts:

1. Statements of why the topic's concepts and skills are worth spending our classroom, clinical, and judgment time.

2. Reasons nurses have unique ways to make a difference in the topic areas being studied. These are stated values on how nurses are needed to adapt and expand clinical judgment for application of the topic to real situations, for collaboration with other health care providers, and for emerging health challenges all over the world.

Nursing education has moved through the years from a medical model to a pathophysiology systems model and then to a patient problems model. This book proposes using concepts as the teaching model. Concepts such as hydration cut across medical diagnoses, body systems, and patient problems. Also, the vocabulary of concepts is not exclusive to any one group. Concept words such as "safety" form a common language for members of the health care team, for other helping professionals, and for lay people. Adding the uniqueness of the nursing role to mastery concepts shows how nursing has unique perspectives based on the nursing process.

One primary aim of thoroughly learning the priorities in a topic's mastery concepts is that students can gain skill and confidence in the "Aha!" experience of synthesis, or linking the known to the unknown. The skill of synthesizing information will form a major part of their clinical judgment in future years in nursing.

This book attempts to illustrate that an emphasis on priority concepts causes all aspects of a nursing program to relate together meaningfully, from the mission statement to course objectives and eventually to testing and clinical evaluation standards. What is being measured in all our nursing education outcome standards is quality of nursing judgment along with the commitment to the business of "real caring" in making a difference in the health of individuals who need nursing care.

Active Participation Exercises:

The exciting "revolution" in nursing education during recent decades is the change of emphasis to active student learning from an emphasis on teaching. This book has multiple active learning exercises for student engagement, refocusing attention, repetition, recall, varied applications, critical thinking, and creativity. The authors encourage teachers to have students use as many senses they can as much as possible.

Rather than long "talking head" lectures, short explanatory content "bytes" can be alternated with active learning exercises.

Reality Based Clinical Experiences

The authors of this book urge that application of essential content and skills involve early and ongoing practical experiences in clinical labs and in actual patient care situations. They state that the types of assignments, time for priority judgments, and collaborative work with others be made as similar as possible to real nursing situations.

Many examples are given of immediately usable skills such as vital signs: how to do them, how to report and document them, and how to progressively increase skill in interpreting the meaning of normal and abnormal.

Other clinical experience success hints given include giving students very specific directions for clinical site dress, protocols, and tasks so that the students have a sense of predictability and ownership of the situation. Also, the authors emphasize bottom line assessment, such as "real time" short assessments of charts and patients rather than long academic care plans. They encourage forming partnerships with health agency nurses so they participate in care with nurses who have various levels of expertise and unique individual abilities.

Empowerment

Empowerment of students includes not only a focus on priority concepts but also forming positive relationships between and among teachers and students. According to the authors of this book, these relationships built on mutual respect and partnership in nursing education can strongly affect learning. All teachers and students have both strengths and frailties. Together their mutual commitment in the teaching-learning partnership can be to apply their growing wisdom and skills to assist other individuals and groups who need the unique helping ways of nursing.

The nursing value of informed caring (whole person nurses caring for whole person patients) can include whole person students and teachers. This means a quality of relationships between and among teachers and students that fosters a strong sense of community. The message "We are in this thing together" is sometimes reserved for the last Senior level nursing courses that emphasize transitions into professional nurse roles.

Student and teacher roles are different from one another. While both roles are useful, the differences between them can only be bridged with frank and sincere respect, not with superficial friendliness pasted over an atmosphere of faculty control and ownership of the total nursing education experience.

Conclusions

Authors Sylvia Rayfield and Loretta Manning have brought alive for us the message that our highest calling as nursing teachers is to develop teaching strategies and relationships with nursing students that foster in them a sense of worth and of identity as caring professional nurses. The dual aims of focus and empowerment have been intended to revolutionize not only the teaching of nursing but nursing teachers themselves. Teachers are urged to find mentors, use resources on teaching, and to trust themselves as caring and expert clinicians. The book has sought to awaken the consciousness of faculty to what nursing education is really all about.

Addendum

One visual picture that has helped the author of this synopsis summarize the wonderful teaching wisdom of this book is that of the three parts of a peacock: head, body, and tail.

Head: The peacock's head represents priority concepts for nursing knowledge, reasoning, critical thinking, rationales, principles, and clinical implications. This area includes active use of our "knower" plus a commitment to progressing increasing our awareness that we "know what we know" related to nursing judgment.

Body: The peacock's body represents active reality-based learning. This is literally the "heart" of learning in an application profession such as nursing. The use of case studies, strong visual props, and memory clues can help tremendously in how student nurses process and apply essential concepts they read in textbooks and hear in the classroom. It empowers them to combine old and new learning. Getting into the habit of active learning can inspire them to make a commitment to a lifelong process of a continual updating of their knowledge and skills.

Tail: The peacock's beautiful tail represents the fabulous "extras" that make current and lifelong learning fascinating. Teachers can use media news and information illustrations as well as health care research to form flashy and memorable "circles" of facts, meanings, and intriguing questions. Taking time to develop a repertoire of skillful teaching strategies involves more than just keeping students awake as teachers make learning exciting and fun. You can also inspire students to become more informed and caring nurses.

Chapter 2

THE PATH OF LEARNING
THROUGH RELATIONSHIPS

"In everyone's life, at some time, our inner fire goes out.
It is then burst into flame by an encounter with another human being.
We should all be thankful for those people who rekindle the inner spirit."
Albert Schweitzer

Many of us have heard this warning given to students in their first lecture in nursing school, "Look to your left, look to your right, only one of you will be here at the end of the semester." I know I received that lecture when I first started nursing school in the 1950s and I know that my young 18 year old cousin got the same speech last year in her first lecture. It's still happening!

One of my closest colleagues had a unique way of starting her students out each semester. She said, "I doubt that you can make any mistake that I have not already made. The difference is, I know how to get out of it. Come to me when you make a mistake and let me help you get out of it."

What a difference there is in the feel of those two statements. Can you get a sense of contrasts in the energy and the atmosphere in those two classrooms? Students learn when they are peaceful and calm and like their instructor. Stress and one-upmanship are definitely detrimental to learning. I've had many instructors over the last years say, "I'm not running a popularity contest. I don't care whether they like me or not." We have found that the more students like their instructor, the more motivated they are to learn.

Some of the most interesting literature and research on this topic that I have read comes from Tim Sanders, writer for the New York Times and leadership coach at Yahoo. Tim is an advocate for good values in business. The research that is quoted in his book, *The Likeability Factor,* indicates that "students who perceive a more positive student-professor relationship and like their professors may be more motivated to learn because the presence of the professor is rewarding to them, and they care more about obtaining the approval of the professor". This finding is helpful. As nursing professors, we need all the help that we can get!

Sanders' book can be summed up in one word, the word **LIKE**. Here is an acronym to help you remember.

LIKE	
L	Listen with empathy. Connect with the students' wants and needs.
I	Invest in relevance. Teach those things that they must know and find useful.
K	Keep friendly. Being unfriendly has been documented as counterproductive in the learning process.
E	Emanate your real self. Friendship and empathy cannot be faked.

What makes a student like their instructor? Sometimes it's the big things and sometimes the little things, but a combination of both is very useful. Big things include **RESPECT** for the student as a human being.

Acronyms are a great way for people to learn and we will use a heap of them in this book. We will also use italics as another way to talk to you.

RESPECT	
R	Reach the students with your eyes when you talk. Look at them and let them know with your look that you care about them. If there are disagreements, approach them with the spirit of resolution.
E	Empower them. This is a whole path in itself and will be spoken about much more later in the book. For now, remember that knowledge is power. Empower them with knowledge.
S	Show them by modeling. Model how to initiate relationships and how to nurture themselves and others. *It's hard to model nurturing yourself when you never take a bathroom or lunch break. We have to show them that we and they are as important as everyone. Hospitals say, "The patient comes first." We believe that if the nurse does not care for her/himself, she/he will not be able to care for the patients.*
P	Practice what you preach. If you tell them that class starts at 8, be there yourself. If you tell them to dress professionally, do so yourself. If you tell them to be gentle and caring with their patients, be gentle and caring with them. If you tell them to study hard to learn, then you study hard to keep current and learn ways to teach so that they can remember.
E	Enlist ownership. Students need input into their learning. In order to enlist their ownership, we need to share expectations. We should ask where they are and what they need.
C	Collaborate with students in their learning and encourage them to collaborate with each other. This is a partnership not a competition.
T	Try loving them and holding high expectations. You will get what you expect as they will rise to the occasion. *As Yoda says,"Don't try, do."*

16

Respect is an excellent way to develop trust between yourself and students. They need that trust. They know that you hold their future in your hands. Be gentle.

Relationships with students are founded on our relationship with ourselves as individuals. How can we respect others if we do not respect ourselves? How do we build a relationship with ourselves? Are we comfortable with our knowledge or are we threatened by questions? Do we have a need to be "in control"? What will make us peaceful? Are we always looking for a reason to be offended? Are we the "watchdog" that says, "If they are going to be a nurse they will have to get by me?" It's our attitude, our comfort in walking in our own shoes that allows us to establish relationships with others.

We believe that it is very hard to respect oneself if one is being abused either verbally or physically. If you find yourself in this situation, remember, you are the only one who can get yourself out of it. A famous quote states, *"If you find yourself in a hole, quit digging."* Certainly do not let any one else dig a hole for you. There are too many resources in this country to live in fear and misery.

We have all observed considerable abuse in nursing schools. Most faculties have agreed with the prevalence of this abuse when we bring it to their attention. For example, what major in the university has the most clock hours for a degree requirement? Which major has to write nursing care plans until 3 o'clock in the morning and when they get to the hospital the next day, their patients have died or been discharged and the nursing care plan that they worked on is now useless? What other student gets a letter stating that even though everyone else is starting the semester on September 1st, all nursing majors, must report on August 15th, for orientation? What other major may be sitting in class at 3 o'clock one afternoon when someone walks in and says, "I want my entire clinical group to stay until 5 this afternoon because we have to get ready to go to the hospital next week"? Often no consideration is given to children, spouses, or other commitments. Who else has several major papers and projects in one semester? Who else must pass a math test with 100% accuracy before they can continue past the first week in their major? Most nursing faculty do not even recognize these practices as being abusive. This is the way that they were treated when they went to nursing school and just believe that it goes with the territory.

Authenticity plays a large part in relationships and respect. I have a wonderful picture of my grandson with a teddy bear that reminds me of the children's story *The Velveteen Rabbit*. As you remember, this story was about a child's favorite stuffed animal that was loved so much it finally became real. *The nursing student needs to see real.* They need to know that you will do what you say that you will do and that this will not change unless you advise them of the change first. A lack of authenticity or honesty is sensed by the student and is very damaging to all relationships.

Relationships are built and enhanced through respectful communication. We are living in such a great age of technology that we can have instant communication at our fingertips. Communication is a way to alleviate fears and a way to make the student more confident. It can be used as a learning strategy in many ways; everything from a copy of map quest that shows them the way to their next clinical assignment, to what to wear to be in compliance with agency dress codes. The content is obviously important in communication, but we believe that the intent and tone of that content will make or break relationships. Caring communication is way at the top of the list for establishing relationships.

We have observed many different kinds of relationships in nursing school. Some of them are based on fear and many of them are based on, "I am the teacher and you are the student and I know what you need." Relationships that nurture are few and far between in many of our nursing programs.

Nathan Schwartz-Salant in *The Mystery of Human Relationship*, summed it up when he said, "Relationships are not only forms of exchange of energy and function between people but also living structures which regulate a person's sense of identity and well-being." All relationships are something that we do! This is exactly the path. *Our highest calling as nursing teachers is to develop relationships with our students that provide them with a feeling of well-being and give them a sense of identity as a caring and compassionate nurse.*

Nothing in relationship building precludes holding the learner accountable or lowering educational standards. We do not "let them slide" or accept a sloppy performance because we want them to like us or because we want a good student evaluation. Learners, like everyone, must know where the boundaries are. They have to know that there are consequences if boundaries are crossed. *Do not avoid disagreements; infuse them with grace and with the spirit reaching a win-win resolution. This provides an environment where students can learn.*

Our belief is: set the boundaries and the goals, point them in the right direction and get out of the way. There is no doubt that something in the relationship between a teacher and a learner enhances the learning process.

As nursing faculty continue on this "path of learning through relationships", we will not only expand our influence, but will inspire our students to be excellent nurses. *The definition of inspire is "to breathe life into another".* Isn't this what relationships are all about? Isn't nursing about this as well? I have outlined below several characteristics that are imperative throughout this process of relationship building with our students.

These are self explanatory, so I will not elaborate on the acronym; however, the bottom line is that it is impossible to breathe life into another if you don't have life in yourself.

INSPIRE	
I	Inner security
N	Nothing is as fast as the speed of TRUST
S	Stretch ourselves to develop skills that will equal the challenges with students
P	Personal moral authority
I	Integrity
R	Relate to self
E	Empathize

"Treat a man as he is and he will remain as he is; treat a man as he can and should be and he will become as he can and should be." These are profound and true words of the poet Goethe.

I had a wonderful opportunity to work with a group of nurse leaders on a book entitled, *The Untold Stories of Nursing*. As I was editing the stories I was impressed with one of the stories written by a nursing student who shares how she was scared when her patient's clinical status started to deteriorate, but due to the confidence that the patient had in her she was able to overcome her fear and assist the patient. She did all the right interventions such as assessment, reporting the findings, repositioning, etc. The patient believed in her as a nurse even while she was studying and preparing for the new role! The patient saw beneath the surface, beyond the obvious. *"The patient entrusted me with her life far beyond my current experience and ability." "I was trusted without evidence and without proof."* The student reported this as a crossroads in her education. What a strong lesson! "The patient believed and knew I would rise to the challenge, treated me accordingly, and I did."

Patricia Thompson, RN, EdD, Sigma Theta Tau International also says it well, *"...Early in my career, I was powerfully influenced by a nursing instructor who saw potential in me that I did not recognize. Under the watchful, yet caring, tutelage of this person, I began to find my professional self."*

In the rapidly changing world of health care, nursing instructors must develop a climate of trust with students, so that students recognize that perfection is an unrealistic expectation, have the courage to ask questions, and feel that they can discuss mistakes when these occur without fear of embarrassment or reprimand. Students must have confidence and trust that the instructor is competent in correcting mistakes and addressing consequences without distressing the patient or undermining the student's confidence.

Trust becomes a verb when you communicate to others their worth and potential so clearly that they are inspired to work hard and to see it in themselves. Trust is also the highest form of motivation. This is what nursing faculty are all about! We serve others, trust others, see their worth and potential and provide opportunity for growth, development, and encouragement. If students do not live true to this trust, then it will deteriorate and they will not be inspired to experience their own worth and potential. This is definitely where we must establish boundaries and standards.

Relationships are all about partnerships. The most beautiful example of this is the true story of Helen Keller and her teacher, Anne Sullivan. Helen Keller was deaf and blind. Anne Sullivan was legally blind herself and had an abusive childhood, but overcame this and was deeply transformed through serving and teaching one student, Helen Keller. The contributions that Helen Keller made have been inspiring, motivating, and never ending. The key to all of this was her teacher! What kind of a teacher are you?

Chapter 3

THE PATH OF LEARNING THROUGH ENGAGEMENT AND EMPOWERMENT

"The best way to inspire people to a superior performance is to convince them by everything you do and by your everyday attitude that you are wholeheartedly supporting them."
Harold H. Greneen, Former Chairman of ITT

In almost every workshop that I have presented, the faculty group has a great concern regarding student motivation. The words that I hear everywhere are, "The students are not like they used to be. The students don't read. The students don't come to class prepared. The students don't come to clinical prepared. The students ..."

For these reasons, faculties want to know how they can motivate the students and they are right. The students do need reasons to be engaged. *If they don't have reasons to learn, we lose them.*

I was recently working with a school that had a 50% pass rate on NCLEX. Faculty members felt that their students were not motivated and were not interested in anything they had to say. I learned that they began their semester the end of August and were not taking students to the clinical agencies until December. My concern is that students were delayed in being able to apply what they were learning.

Most nursing students come to nursing school because they want to help people. They want to wear that uniform and go to the hospital. We can use that motivation if we don't kill it at the start. If they have to go to endless classes on philosophy and have tests on Florence Nightingale, (primary, secondary and tertiary), they lose the motivation that they have when they come in.

How do we keep that? One of the most important parts of the first semester is the Fundamentals Lab. You can call it Introduction to Nursing, Basic Laboratory, Skills Lab or whatever, but what it amounts to are Fundamentals, things that students need to know to care for patients. This is where we can enhance that motivation. I say enhance, because I don't believe that we can motivate anyone, I think that motivation comes from inside. I do certainly believe that we can enhance their motivation.

One of the ways to enhance their motivation is to get them into hospitals and other clinical settings as student nurses just as soon as possible. "As soon as possible" is certainly relative, especially among programs that are having problems with motivation. What we are really doing in those first few days is setting values. That which we teach first must be very important, so let's use those first few days and weeks to our advantage and theirs. The first week can be used to teach universal precautions and hand washing. Why start there? How many of us have taken our first clinical group to the hospital for the first time, paused on the hospital steps and prayed, "God, just don't let them kill anybody today!" The way they can kill someone in that first trip to the hospital is to walk from patient to patient without washing their hands!

Why does our nosocomial infection rate keep rising? We believe one reason is that nurses and other health care workers do not have hand washing as a value. We as faculty can begin to make that change, we can teach it first so that the students know that it is a value.

Another value for that first week is the student's observational skills. This can be taught using the nursing process. Some faculty groups get hung up on nursing process and take two to three weeks to teach it. They write questions for exams that ask, "What part of the nursing process is this or that?" We believe that the more the student uses the nursing process the better their observational skills will be and they will innately learn which is which. *It is hard for the student to learn and remember if they can't figure out a way to use the process. If it cannot be used, why are you teaching it?*

It is hard for the student to assess if they do not at least have one usable tool. One primary tool is the skill to take vital signs. This skill can be taught in the first week of fundamentals lab along with universal precautions and hand washing. Teach them how to do TPR and blood pressure and assess for pain during that first lab week. Then the second week of the semester, take them to the hospital to do assessments with vital signs just for a couple of hours. For another couple of hours take them to the nursing home to do assessments and vital signs. For another couple of hours take them to the day nursery to do assessments and vital signs. For one more session, take them to the shopping mall to do assessments and vital signs. FREE BLOOD PRESSURES TAKEN HERE! We want them to take so many blood pressures that their ears rise, yet they know which size cuff to use on which arm, how to approach people to begin relationships, how to assess pain on patients of all ages and how to gain confidence with their assessment abilities. ALL done within the first two weeks of school. This is an action that motivates. It makes them feel that they belong and that they are doing something. They are being a nurse and are doing things that "lay people" cannot do. They have a secret of their own even if it's just how to take vital signs.

Wilson's (1994) qualitative study of baccalaureate nursing students in a senior-level clinical course reports that students tend to equate learning with the first-time performance or mastery of a growing list of psychomotor skills. Students seem unable to concentrate on the larger patient care situation until they feel comfortable with the hands-on-care they are providing. This focus on skilled clinical performance in accomplishing patient care procedures is likely to be related to the goal of looking good as a nurse.

Focusing on a list of skills appropriate to the setting, the instructor is able to satisfy the need students have to develop clinical expertise through technical skill performance.

Students routinely report that once they feel confident with their hands then they can concentrate on their head which includes the critical thinking that correlates with the procedure or skill.

We must begin teaching critical thinking and clinical reasoning on day one. That means we cannot just teach the skill of taking blood pressures and vital signs. We have to teach the normal range of these skills and what they should do as a second week freshman nursing student if they assess signs outside the normal range. We also need to teach them in the lab how to document these vital signs. We can use hospital flow sheets and show them how to record their findings. We have now started their learning on another value. "If you didn't chart it, you didn't do it".

There are several things that a nursing instructor can do to make these first couple of weeks easy, exciting and non-stressful. We call them the **"W's"**.

THE W's
What to wear, what the dress code is for a nursing student to go to the hospital agency or represent the college at the mall.
What to bring. Do they need their own blood pressure cuffs, bandage scissors, hospital ID?
What time to be there. They will learn to plan. (Part of the nursing process.)
Where to park. It's hard to think when the City's finest is towing your car.
Which unit to get to and how to get there. There may be 3 units on 3rd floor.
What time they will plan to leave for their post class or home.
Where they can find you. You are their life line.

These "**W's**" lessen anxiety, provide information and help them belong. Their ability to approach a patient, assess vital signs, document the information, share the information if necessary, and get safely back home is empowering. They can't help but be engaged, because they are being nursing students! They need that empowerment because it will engage them, and they need it early in the nursing program.

This same logic brings us to recommend teaching CPR in the first semester. I know you're asking why. Here's the path. *We want to prepare them for the worst thing that can ever happen to them so that they will be empowered.* What is worse than someone dying and not knowing what to do? If we will teach emergency procedures early, they will be empowered and have a sense of security. We must teach that we will not save everyone with CPR, but we at least know what to do and will do the best that we can. I can hear some of you now saying, "The first semester is way too early to teach CPR." Just remember that lay people take CPR and they are not nursing students. There are no prerequisites to basic CPR. *Empower them.*

You have set a precedent with this first couple of weeks. Plan that first semester with care so that a nursing concept is taught one day and is being practiced the next day. Repetition is the mother of learning. Let them see it, hear it, think about it, practice it and then **DO IT**. Choose carefully and prioritize the concepts in the first semester. Yes, physical assessment has to be a big part of early student learning in nursing.

Our experience indicates that the student is taken to the hospital only after having completed several classes in physical assessment. They are often given a 21 page form to fill out. You can forget seeing them for the rest of the day! I think we do the new nurses a disservice by forcing or allowing them this type of practice. Think about how much time you have to go in and do an assessment of a hospital client. You're lucky if you have 2-3 minutes! Why should we teach new students to take hours to fill out a 21 page form? They never do it this way in reality.

How can we teach assessment without going through this process? We have to teach them to prioritize. Except for admissions, a nurse rarely gets to spend very much time doing an assessment so we can teach system specific assessment and help them with time management. If we don't start time management on day one, they will take 15 minutes to wash their hands. Of course if we don't give them some sense of time, they may take five seconds to wash their hands.

One of my favorite techniques to teach assessment is to line up an entire clinical group, arrange for them to be in front of me one at the time at 10 minute intervals. Send the first one to a room down the hall and tell them to come back in five minutes and tell me what they see. I start off with asking the student, what did you see?

They usually start off with, "There's a woman in the bed.

Anyone else in the room?

Yea, there's a guy sitting in the chair at the end of the bed.

Significant other?

UH...

Did they have an IV running?

Yea, I say one of those machines. (IVAC)

What medications were in the IV?

UH...

How much fluid was left in the IV?

UH...

Did they have a Foley catheter?

Yes, I saw the catheter bag.

How much fluid was in the bag?

UH...

Was there a wheelchair in the room?

Yes, there was a wheelchair beside the bed.

Were the big wheels in the front or the back?
UH......

By this time, they are aware that their observational and assessment skills are somewhat lacking. What is so amazing is that by the time I ask the same questions to the last student in the group, they will have all the answers even to "The big wheels are in the back!!!!"

It's fun to see learning take place. Notice that I did not say to the first student, "Don't tell the other students what I am asking." This leads to game playing. *We don't care how they learn, just that they learn.* We want them to learn in a timely fashion. They are going to have to practice in a timely fashion once they become clinicians.

If we do not teach them how to do things in a timely manner, they are so disillusioned when they graduate and go into practice that many of them quit within the first 2 years. They feel guilty about not getting everything done. *One of our paths is to teach the learner to prioritize and to feel good about what they have gotten done, not bad about what they did not get done.*

Engagement and empowerment are two of the most important paths that we can take. We have to determine how to use them throughout the entire teaching-learning program.

The result will be students who exhibit self-control, self-management and are self-organizing. These students will have a **DEEP** desire to be an outstanding nurse.

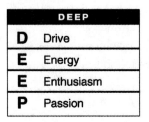

DEEP	
D	Drive
E	Energy
E	Enthusiasm
P	Passion

The roots of the word enthusiasm mean "God in you." Empowerment is exactly the same thing, only it is the students having the knowledge to do the work they love and doing it in a way that meets their deepest needs and the priority needs of the patient. Isn't this the outcome we want from nursing education?

Chapter 4

THE PATH OF LEARNING THROUGH COLLABORATION

"The purpose of life is to live it, to taste experience to the utmost, to reach out eagerly and without fear for newer and richer experience."
Eleanor Roosevelt

For years students have always wanted to choose their own clinical groups. Faculties have resisted this request because they do not want the students to "get dependent on each other". In fact, some faculty have been particularly controlling. Even though the students may live in the same town, 50 miles from the agency and have wanted to coordinate their transportation, faculty would not let them be in the same clinical group.

We believe that the desire to work together should be used to advantage. *The principle here is that he who teaches learns the most.* For this reason, we should not be worried about people being in the same clinical group for more than one semester. We have found that students who stay in the same clinical group all the way through school help each other grow, become accountable, cover one another's backs and develop a sense of loyalty and team.

Collaboration is a powerful secret of teaching. At the top of the list is collaboration with the instructor. *Collaboration precludes the one up and one down position as it gives a feeling that we are in this together.* We believe that this is one of the most powerful concepts in nursing education. This is not a competition. I am not out to get you. I am here to help you learn and to learn from you. *We are in this together!*

There are many ways to foster collaboration. These are suggestions that can be used sporadically or all the time and still be effective. For example, for a unit test:

- Divide the students into groups of three.

- Give each of them an answer sheet and let them collaborate on the answers on the test. Remember each one has an answer sheet and each will get a separate grade. They do not have to agree with the consensus of the group, but can still maintain their answer if they are adamant.

- Each person submits their own answer sheet and gets their grade based on their thinking. There is an amazing amount of learning that takes place using this collaboration. One of the side effects is that it takes longer to take this kind of exam due to the amount of discussion and learning that is taking place. For this reason the exam should be somewhat shorter than an exam that is used without collaboration.

Many of us have used joint assignments especially on special projects. Our own experience and the experience of current students say that one person often does all of the work and others get the grade setting up an unfair situation in the student's mind. For this reason, we have found it better to do collaboration, especially on unannounced exams. The collaboration happens, the learning takes place, but no one depends on another for preparation of the exam. Special projects deserve a mention of their own and will be discussed in the chapter regarding assignments.

There are many other ways to set up collaboration, especially in clinical assignments. Some faculty get hung up on every student having their own patient and being responsible for total patient care. We have learned that students learn from each other when they collaborate on the same patient. This is especially true when the students are not on the same academic level. The freshmen learn confidence and how to establish relationships from the seniors and the seniors learn how to teach and develop their future staff by working with the younger students. These are just a few of the interactions that take place.

- Collaborative teaching works great in a classroom regardless of the number of students in the class. We use a technique called "Choose A Partner". You have 20 seconds to choose a partner from someone sitting on a different row than yours. Make a decision which one will be A and which one will be B. We give them about 30 seconds (it takes 10 seconds for what you've said to sink in) and then ask for a show of hands for all of the A's and then a show of hands for the B's. This gets engagement, participation and changes the energy in the room. Then we use something that we need for them to review or learn as the subject, such as CPR.
- The A's have 2 minutes to write everything they know about CPR in the adults.
- The B's have 2 minutes to write everything they know about CPR

in babies and neonates.

- At the end of 2 minutes (earlier if they start getting talkative) tell them that A has one minute to tell B everything they know about CPR in the adult, but remember we are in this together so if A happens to leave anything our then B fills in what they remember.

- After one minute call time and tell B that they have one minute to tell A everything they know about CPR in babies, but again remember that we are in this together so A will fill in anything that is missed.

- All in all, this exercise takes about five minutes. Their brain has been working, they have participated and collaborated and you, the instructor, have kept your mouth shut except for timekeeping.

Sometimes we as faculty get to the point of thinking, "If it doesn't come out of my mouth, it has not been taught." Wrong. Collaboration is very powerful because learners are teaching each other. Please do not go back now and reteach CPR after this exercise, because the students need to know that what is in their brain is just as important as what is in yours.

Collaboration leads to learning from mistakes with fewer traumas. It provides a safe environment for students to learn. The attitude of collaboration and *we are in this together* increases the confidence level of the student and decreases their stress level. Stress is a robber of confidence. We want to do all that we can to provide an atmosphere of calm and competence.

Not only have we found this strategy to be very effective both in clinical as well as the classroom setting, but collaborative learning success has been documented through research at Stanford, the University of Minnesota, and in numerous nursing journal articles.

Collaboration assists in focusing the student's minds on what they know and on what you want them to know. This will also motivate them to listen with that purpose in mind. As Abigail Van Buren stated, *"The less you talk, the more you're listened to."* I don't know about you, but I enjoy having a few minutes of silence while the class is working together and better yet, the learning outcomes are great! In this Information Age, can we afford or do we have the time to keep our students in isolation in the learning environment anymore? When we are resuscitating a patient in the ICU, does a successful outcome depend on working in isolation? When we manage or lead a group of nurses, do we work in isolation? Collaboration is indeed a conduit to success for learning, clinical practice, and leadership. This conduit will assist the students in having the confidence to know they CAN do it!

Chapter 5

THE PATH OF LEARNING WITH OWNERSHIP

"Life isn't about finding yourself. Life is about creating yourself."
Unknown

Years ago, I went to a university to present a follow-up faculty development workshop. When I arrived at the airport, the Dean of Nursing met me to take me to my hotel. She gave me the local newspaper and asked me to read the headline. It said, "NURSING FACULTY RESIGNS." I asked her what happened. She asked if I remembered the assignment that I had suggested to them on my last consultation. Of course I did. They had told me that they had a 55% NCLEX pass rate and were going to be closed by the board of nursing if they did not have at least an 85% pass rate with their next graduating class. I taught them how to write clinical reasoning questions as they are reflected on the NCLEX and suggested that they utilize an exit exam for this class until we had time to work on the curriculum issues. They told me that they had 12 students that would never pass. I suggested that they write these 12 names on a piece of paper and see if their intuition was accurate. They rewrote their exams with a higher difficulty level and administered the exit exam. Exactly 12 people out of a class of 50 failed the exam. Yes, they were the same 12 students that the faculty had written on their list. *Intuition is highly accurate and is a direct line of communication from the Divine.*

They gave the 12 students an F in the class and passed the rest, now confident that they were graduating competent nurses that could pass the NCLEX. They submitted their grades to the academic vice president who thought that this was a pretty high failure rate in the last semester and decided to run it by the board. One of the 12 that had been unsuccessful was the granddaughter of the chairman of the board of the university. You can probably guess the rest. The chairman said, "My granddaughter is not going to be the victim of an experimental program!" He ordered the president to change all of the failing grades to a pass so that all students would graduate. Hence the headline, NURSING FACULTY RESIGNS. This was the Sunday paper and I was there to do a curriculum revision workshop on

Monday for the three faculty that were left.

Here is where I got caught in my own omnipotence. I thought I could carry it off! I did not ask them about what they wanted to talk about, or what they needed to learn from me. I gave them no ownership. I just went right on with my planned agenda. By the first break, I knew what a terrible mistake that I was making. The three faculty members that were left were feeling terribly guilty because they had not resigned. They felt their principles and professionalism had been questioned. They wanted to quit, but were caught with being the only bread winner in the families. How indeed could they hear about curriculum revision? This is a unique situation, but it sure drilled into my head that *we should never go into a room with a planned agenda or content without first asking the learners what they need to learn.*

We begin every class with "shared expectations". This is an exercise that asks the learner what they need to hear from us today. Granted, they may say, "You're the teacher, we're paying you to tell us what we need to know." Sound familiar? The point is, most of them have not read and have no idea what is scheduled in today's content.

One of the ways to get them engaged is to tell them that tomorrow in clinical they may be assigned a client that has difficulty breathing. What additional assessments do they need to make? Is the client receiving blood? IV fluids? Any medications? What do they need to know about how to care for this client? I assure you, it is **not** how to do a bed and bath. Start with empowering them with what to do first. They can roll up the head of the bed and begin oxygen immediately. Does the client need lasix from orders on protocol for fluid overload? It's amazing how wonderful it is to have something to do when you know your client is in distress. Yes, of course, this is just a start. Now we have to continue to assess and determine what else they need to know. This leads us to the next chapter on how to prioritize the content of a class.

In closing this chapter, our role as educators is not to fill their box with every detail known to nursing because, as we know, just when we think we have a handle on information it changes! *Our role is to light their fire from within!* We need to inspire them to take ownership of their educational process. This process of learning has only just begun in school!

As partners in this learning process, we have an exciting responsibility to lead, facilitate and motivate the students' growth and development into professional nurses. It is an honor for us to be part of such an influential time in the student's life and to have the privilege to begin this path with them and inspire each student we teach to continue this path for a lifetime! As we tell students and graduates in our workshops, the key to success is not only having the correct answer but being able to ask the best questions. We intentionally positively reinforce students when they display the courage to ask questions in class or in clinical that reflect critical thinking. This is one way that we know we are partners on the *"path of learning with ownership."* What do you do as an educator to guide the students down this path? What do you currently do to inspire the student to LEARN?

LEARN
L   Learner feels the need to learn
E   Espouse the goals of learning as their own (students)
A   Active in the learning process
R   Responsibility is shared for planning and implementing the learning experience
N   Nurturing environment conducive for trust, **respect**, and helpfulness assisting progress toward learning goals

"LEARN" was adapted from Knowles (1980) research proposing ideal conditions under which adults learn best.

Chapter 6

THE PATH OF PRIORITIZING CONTENT FOR PRESENTATION

"Other people may be there to help us, teach us,
Guide us along our path.
But the lesson to be learned is always ours."
Melody Beattie

Many course syllabi have chapter and page numbers that will be "covered" on a specific class day. Typically, the faculty member hauls out the Power Point, outlines the chapter starting on page 1, posts the notes on Blackboard and "lectures" on the chapter content.

How can we expect our students to prioritize if we do not prioritize ourselves? Here is a method of prioritizing content that leads to understanding and empowering the student. What if your chapter is 100 pages long and you have one hour to "lecture" on it? Please do not outline the chapter. Just because it is outlined on Power Point does not mean it is prioritized. Say to yourself, "If I only had one thing that I could tell the learner about this content, what would it be?" Now that I have identified THE thing that they must remember, how am I going to help them remember it?

We know that the vast majority of learners think and learn in images. Use this example on your students. "I am going to say a word and I want you to tell me what you see in your head." (Now you have their attention, they will all participate) "The word is elephant. What do you see?" Many of them will say "trunk, tail, big, gray" or other words that describe an elephant. Then you ask the question, "How many of you saw the word elephant written across your brain?" Depending on the number in the class you may have 0-4 that will raise their hand. Your next comment is, "We know that we think and learn in images and we will use images to help you remember things." This demonstration gets the learner to participate and realize the power of an image in learning.

Who comes up with the images that can be used for learners? ICAN Publishing Inc. has two books, *Nursing Made Insanely Easy* and *Pharmacology Made Insanely Easy,* that have some excellent images that you may want to use in your class. These books are sold on the international market and can be ordered through http://www.icanpublishing.com. If these books do not have an image that is suitable for your use, make one up. The funnier the image, the better. You don't have to be an artist, use stick figures. That is how the authors of the "Made Easy" books started. The objective is to provide an image that will give the learner a way to think about the concept that you are teaching.

Let me give you an example. Here is a picture of Cushy Carl.

CUSHY CARL

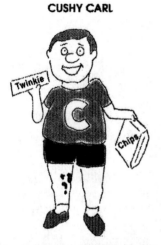

Cushy either has Cushing's disease or is taking corticosteroid drugs. In one hand, he is holding chips. What do we know about chips? They are salty. If Cushy is holding salt he is also holding water because salt draws water to it. If he is holding water he is holding both volume and pressure. This will cause him to weigh more and have a tendency toward hypertension. In his other hand he is holding a Twinkie. Twinkies are dessert cakes that are full of sugar. If Cushy is holding sugar then his blood sugar level is increased (hyperglycemia). Look at his leg and see a sore that will not heal because his blood sugar is so high. He also has a moon face and a buffalo hump. This is a typical picture of clients taking corticosteroid drugs for a long length of time.

With this explanation the learner has a way of thinking about Cushing's syndrome or steroid drugs and their effects on clients. *The picture is so unique that will students will remember it and be able to think about questions or clinical situations that relate to it.* Using an image is just one way to move things from the learners very short term memory to long term memory.

There are many paths to prioritizing content. We want our learners to be safe. We have used the acronym SAFETY to help you prioritize the content that you are preparing to teach.

SAFETY

S The **S** stands for <u>system specific assessment</u>. This skill is high on the priority list for assessment to determine what issues the client is presenting. For example, learners do not have time to complete a full physical assessment if the client is having chest pain; therefore, they must be taught to complete a fast cardiac/lung assessment. System specific assessment must be applied to clinical safety. Learners do not make this jump in cognition unless the instructor teaches it in every unit and then practices it every clinical day. *How can we empower the learner if we don't show them how to look for what is going on?* We want them to think "assess" from the minute the overhead light comes on and they walk in the door of the client's room.

A The **A** stands for <u>accuracy of orders and assignments</u>. We want the student to think about the provider's orders and decide if the orders are accurate. Yes, they are ordered, but do we want to carry that order out? Do we really want to give that much Morphine? Is the client terminal? Does the order match the client assessment?
Students must be taught whether to accept and how to make assignments from an early date in the curriculum. Part of their being safe is determined by their acceptance of an assignment that is given to them.
As leaders, they will be expected to assign clients to different levels of health care workers. How can they make these assignments if they do not know the scope of practice of all health care workers?

F The **F** in safety stands for <u>firsts</u>. What actions do we accomplish first? How do we prioritize whether this client should be seen before another client? How do we prioritize which nursing action that we complete on this particular client before we do anything else? Sometimes there may be 10 things to do. We have to empower them by helping them learn priorities.

E This **E** is a biggie. It is <u>evaluating pharmacology</u>. This includes evaluating the correct dose and all of the other "rights" of medication administration. It also includes determining the rationale for the client receiving this drug; the drugs effect on the client; drug/drug interaction; and drug/food interaction. How can the client live taking this drug for the rest of their life? What blood tests must they have and how often? How do the results of these blood levels affect the actions of nurses? As we know, many symptoms and findings from system specific physical assessment are medication related. All "medication" is not prescribed. Clients have a propensity for picking up "supplements" at the health food store, having no idea that it may react with their coumadin or other drugs that they have been prescribed. Due to the numerous drug/drug interactions, food/drug interactions, the many issues with polypharmacy with the older client, I CAN Publishing, Inc. has developed a one day Pharmacology Made Insanely Easy Course (http://www.icanpublishing.com). Many schools of nursing are incorporating this one day course into their curriculum to complement their current pharmacology courses. The students leave being excited about pharmacology! Can you believe this? Come and see for yourself! *There is nothing more energizing and transforming than when you can remember concepts, apply them, and know the questions to ask!*

T The **T** stands for Teach and Test infection control. We have to set this value in our first week of teaching. We set it in the skills lab, in our expectations and by modeling. This sounds like "old hat". If it's so old hat, why are there so many nosocomial infections in the hospital?

Y The **Y** is a bit bold. It stands for CYA (Cover Your Assets). What assets are those? They are things like your nursing license, your financial assets and personal possessions as well as your client's safety. We have to teach our students how to protect themselves and their clients in a litigious society. For example, we must learn about protecting ourselves and clients from confidentiality issues, incompetent, unskilled, intoxicated or drugged staff, unsafe equipment, falls or other injuries in our health care agencies.
These are all areas of personal safety that are high on our priority list and the acronym of SAFETY will help you remember them yourself. This acronym can easily be used as a blueprint for writing and prioritizing you class presentation.

There is another very valuable way to prioritize content and that is by teaching conceptually. Recently, I was presenting a workshop on Teaching Strategies when a young new faculty presented this question. "I have one hour to teach Diabetes Mellitus. How in the world do I cover all of Diabetes in one hour and prioritize it?" My answer is to start by renaming you content to "Hyper and Hypoglycemia".

Many of our nursing curricula are organized around the medical model of cardiac, respiratory, endocrine, and other systems. This is not a bad way to organize, but if we can teach the content in a conceptual way, the learner remembers it and can apply it to other situations. If we teach the concept of hyperglycemia, we can discuss diabetes, Cushing's, Total Parenteral Nutrition, Corticosteroid drugs etc. The learners will recognize hyper and hypoglycemia wherever they see it. They will know what assessments to make, how to determine the accuracy of orders, how to prioritize their actions, how to evaluate pharmacology, how to teach infection control and protect their clients from falls, unsafe staff and poor equipment.

Yes, all of this can be completed in one hour and we have taught much more than Diabetes Mellitus. *Prioritize, Prioritize*. The most important thing is that the learner will have learned in a way that they can apply the content to many different situations.

To show you how important images are in teaching, here are another couple of images that can be used when teaching hypoglycemia.

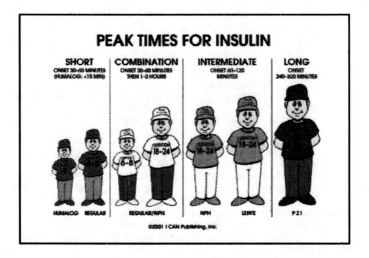

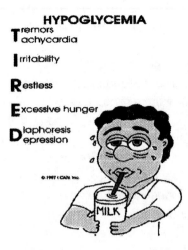

All three of these images come from *Nursing Made Insanely Easy, 4th edition,* Sylvia Rayfield and Loretta Manning. ICAN Publishing. ISBN#0-9643622-8-7. This book and our *Pharmacology Made Insanely Easy* are full of wonderful pictures and bottom line information to help your students learn easily and remember "forever". For further information contact www.icanpublishing.com.

To summarize our priorities, we as faculty have to determine what the priorities are. Students do not have the sophistication or organizational abilities to know what is most important. They certainly will not read before they come to class. We cannot expect them to learn how to prioritize if we cannot present the content in way that makes sense and is usable. Nursing students are adult learners. They don't have time to learn stuff that they can't use. Make the content come alive for them utilizing SAFETY, images and concepts. They will fight to get to your class on time because they will be afraid that they will miss something.

We want to discuss a few no-nos. *You cannot teach the content in a meaningful and memorable way unless you know it yourself.* No-No number 1 for this chapter is the advice to stop using another persons notes. Chances are they outlined the chapter anyway. Now you know how to use images, concepts and SAFETY to prioritize the content in a much better way.

The next path in this chapter can be put into one work SIMPLIFY. *Make the complicated simple is one of the most important concepts in teaching anything.* Many books are on the market with the words simple, easy, and written for those with limited knowledge. All of these indicate how important it is to simplify the complicated. Let me give you an example.

This example is on the concept of fluid overload. Many faculty members hate to teach the concept of fluid and electrolytes because it is a complicated concept. Usually there is one faculty member that has the lecture down pat and if by any chance she has to be absent, the entire schedule will be rearranged so that this can be taught when she gets back, because no one else wants to tackle it. Many times, it's because no one else knows or understands it in a way that they can get it across.

We all know that the student will not read before they come to class so we have to start where they are. This, of course, is one of the main principles of teaching. Let's start with something that they know. Everyone knows what a five gallon paint bucket looks like, so here is an example using something that they know to help them learn a concept that they don't know.

I am holding one five gallon paint bucket in each hand. One of them is full of water; the other is about 2/3 full of water which is similar to our body's fluid level. What if I put the buckets on a scale? Which bucket would weigh the most? The full one, of course. When a body has more fluid in it than it is supposed to have it is called fluid overload. Since we cannot see into the body, we can weigh it to determine if fluid is accumulating. We weigh it at the same time every morning with the same amount of clothes, so that we can get an accurate "daily weight". There is an old saying, "A quart a pound the whole world around." In other words, if the client weighs a pound more that he did yesterday, chances are he has another quart of fluid on board than he had yesterday.

Weight is not the only way to assess extra fluid in the body. The extra fluid has to go somewhere so we as nurses need to look for it. Probably our priority assessment is to look in the lungs, because fluid in the lungs is going to cause our client to be short of breath, become congested and eventually die. Since we can't see in the lungs, we can assess by using our stethoscope to listen. If there is fluid in the lungs we will hear noises (rales and rhonchi) or sounds like the snap, crackle and pop of rice krispies. Yes, they will drown in their own fluid, so the least we can do is sit them up in high fowlers position so that gravity will hopefully pull the fluid to a lower place in the body. The fluid is still there if we can see it pitting in on their legs on in their buttocks, but it is not as death producing in those areas as it is in the lungs.

How do we get rid of this fluid? This is where pharmacology comes in. The client will likely be prescribed a loop diuretic that will cause the body to dump extra fluid into the toilet through the kidneys. How do we know this drug is working? We start by listening again to those lungs and see if the loud crackle lung sounds have decreased and the client is no longer short of breath. We measure intake and output to determine that the output has increased from normal. We also of course weigh the client to see if they have lost that fluid. As you can see, the priority here is not the daily weight, but listening to the lungs for air exchange and assessing the client's clinical picture for decreased shortness of breath.

Before we put these five gallon buckets down, let's put one on each of your feet. Not comfortable right? Which one of these exerts the greatest pressure on your foot? The full one of course. It is easy to see that fluid overload also causes increased pressure, increased blood pressure. So now we have an additional assessment to make. We should be measuring this client's blood pressure as a decrease in fluid volume will also lead to a decrease in blood pressure. Wow! Now you have introduced a whole other concept, fluid volume and hypertension. *The best path of all is tying one concept that the learner understands to a new concept that they need to learn.* You can easily see that you can tie hypertension to the buckets and fluid overload.

We have another concept that can easily be tied in here and that is the fact that potassium will be wasted with loop diuretics. We can bring in laboratory results and what to do when the K is 2.5 or 6.0, again empowering the learner. We can also include concepts that should be taught to the client such as foods that are high in potassium and other drugs that may have an affect on the K level. The learning just keeps going on and on all because they knew about five gallon buckets!

In this example, we are again keeping in mind the SAFETY guidelines, because we're starting with system specific physical assessment, first priorities and evaluating pharmacology. The other concepts in SAFETY can easily be woven into the content to give the learner a bigger overall picture.

Some people think that teaching is one big secret. It is not. All of these are principles of learning found in any good principles of teaching course.

Let us use the word SECRETS to help us remember and sum up these important concepts.

SECRETS	
S	Start where the learner is and know that they won't prepare or read ahead of time
E	Elicit the use of images to increase memory
C	Connect a new concept to one that the learner already knows
R	Remember to simplify the concept from the complicated
E	Empower the learner with actions to increase the clients' well being
T	Teach concepts rather than disease processes
S	SAFETY can be utilized to help you prioritize your teaching content.

"Making the simple complicated is commonplace; making the complicated simple, awesomely simple, that is creativity!"
Charles Mingus, (legendary jazz musician)

Chapter 7

PATHWAYS OF UTILIZING TECHNOLOGY IN NURSING EDUCATION

Darlene Franklin, RN, MSN

Technology—What a scary sounding word, at least to those of us born before the Nintendo Era. As nurse educators we are required to be somewhat up to date with computer technology, but so many of us muddle about wondering when the madness will stop. Remember the first time you used a word processor? What about the frustrations you experienced changing from one word processing package to another? And worst of all, the terror and heartache of a computer crash or meltdown? Sometimes technology is our best friend and on occasion our greatest foe.

But, remember when you mastered the word processor, and when you successfully sent your first email to the other side of the world in a flash. These are the times you felt empowered, the times you discovered you could use technology without knowing all the intricate workings of the computer or the Internet. These were the moments you experienced a transformation—a realization that you were no longer bound by pencil and paper: You were freed by technology to quickly communicate with colleagues, students, and family by clicking. You could store volumes of information on the hard drive, floppy disc, CD, and now the tiny yet mighty, flashdrive/thumbdrive. Technology empowers you to do more in less time. These were the times technology transported you down new and exciting pathways.

How can we use technology to increase student and program outcomes while decreasing faculty workload? What commonly encountered problems in traditional nursing education can be improved by technology?

Problems Encountered

Nursing faculty use multiple methods of determining what concepts are most important for students to learn. This book covers many of these strategies. Although teachers are more adept at determining the course content, students know best how they learn (Banta, 1995). The Nintendo generation requires multiple stimuli to process and retain information. Repetition is well known for assisting students in retention of data, but there is little time to cover the basics much less time for repetition in the classroom. Students may look at their fifty pound textbooks, feel overwhelmed, and soon realize that reading assignments are impossible to complete before class, if ever. Students expect that a faculty delivered lecture will cover the most important content and that memorization of this information is sufficient for success. Nursing faculty know this strategy is inadequate. It is a game of teach and tell—you teach me what I need to know and I will tell it back to you on the test. Historically, this test preparation strategy worked in secondary and many post-secondary school courses. However, student complaints emerge early, usually after the first nursing exam, and test questions are frequently referred to as "different" and "tricky."

The truth is that nursing tests are different because they are developed to prepare graduates for clinical nursing practice, decision-making, and passage of the *National State Board of Nursing Licensure Exam for Registered Nurses NCLEX-RN™* . Each NCLEX question requires students to make decisions based on multiple concepts using higher levels of Bloom's Taxonomy (Bloom, et.al., 1956) not merely knowledge and comprehension; i.e., lower cognition levels where memorization of material often results in high test scores. Unfortunately, we as nurse educators quickly realize that the teach and tell method of preparing nurses for practice is ineffective and often creates conflict between the faculty/test-writer and student/test-taker. Such encounters interfere with the development of a healthy faculty-student relationship, thus impairing the learning experience. So what other teaching methods can we use to empower students to understand, apply, analyze, synthesize, and evaluate (Bloom, et.al., 1956) concepts of nursing practice that will ultimately improve patient outcomes? What can we do to structure an environment that promotes learning rather than chaos?

The Journey

Technological advancements provide the vehicle for improving learning experiences and an opportunity for us, as faculty, to model our value of lifelong learning by admitting what we do not know and finding and utilizing reputable resources—both literary and human, to assist us in our own learning journey. Today's students frequently know more about technology than does the teacher. How many occasions have you found a young college student helping you to access or set up the technology needed for your class? We must admit it; the Nintendo generation is experienced with using and experimenting with technology. These students and young faculty developed along with technology and continue to use it for instant messaging, downloading music, playing games, and learning. Why, therefore, would we exclude this coping and learning mechanism from nursing education? Why would we not value a technologically experienced young faculty who may need mentoring regarding nursing education but who may be our greatest resource in how to use technology to enhance learning?

The goal of this chapter is to serve as the impetus for a transformation of traditional teaching of both seasoned and technologically literate faculty and for empowering them to use technology beyond merely a communication modem or information storage system. Are you ready for the ride? Put on your seatbelt because what we are about to explore will increase student satisfaction, as well as individual student and program outcomes while decreasing your workload. Sounds like a dream?

Key Relationships: The Secret to Technological Success

Recently, I was coerced into using a new computer *Motion Tablet* with the agreement that I would fulfill some small but significant requirements—primarily to increase use of online teaching. I was hesitant to commit because the contract contained technological activities requiring abilities I did not possess. Reluctantly, I signed the dotted line. Who could refuse such a dangling carrot—free access to the latest technology. I conceded to the requirements and mentally planned how I would accomplish what seemed to be a monumental task.

New technology is wonderful, but if you do not know how to operate it, it is useless. Amazingly, in only one month I had completed almost all the contractual requirements. How? I was set up to succeed—a phenomenon that more frequently occurs in reverse. I was provided in-class learning time and an individual mentor. I was required to meet with my assigned mentor one hour every week. I recall thinking, "Why is so much individual time required? What will we talk about?" In retrospect I find that one hour is insufficient when your mentor values your assets and contributions and is eager to help you use those attributes to improve teaching in your specialty area. I tell my mentor what I need and want, and he transforms my fantasies into technological realities.

Unfortunately, I failed to realize how technology could improve my teaching performance until I was pushed outside my comfort zone. I am now enlightened. How can you get this kind of support?

- *Pathway to Technology Number 1*: **Initiate and establish a good rapport and working relationship with your institution's technology department [ITD].** When you begin utilizing technology beyond your comfort zone, you will need someone you can contact 24/7. It is not unusual to contact your ITD two or three times a week and sometimes two to three times a day as you are learning. Strive to develop close relationships with your ITD colleagues. Survival and success depends on this bond. In nursing terms, a good rapport with your ITD is your technological *Airway*.

- *Pathway to Technology Number 2*: **Find a mentor, someone who is eager to help you use new technology and who keeps abreast of the best software and technological advancements.** This person may exist in your ITD, on your nursing faculty, or in another department on campus. As nurses, we are constantly updating ourselves with the ever changing medical, nursing, and pharmacological advancements, allowing little or no time to follow the evolution of technology. A good mentor sifts through technological innovations and keeps you informed and updated on the information best suited to your teaching style and your students' needs. The empowering and creative mentor enjoys implementation of the latest developments and is eager to assist you in the application and utility of these updates. I talk to my mentor daily. His phone numbers are at the top of my cell phone's quick contact list. Select a mentor who believes in you. In nursing terms—your mentor keeps you Breathing with adequate ventilation and a technological oxygen saturation of 95-100%

- *Pathway to Technology Number 3*: **Use your newly acquired technology as quickly and as frequently as possible.** As we educators know from experience, repetition is a major key to developing competence. Ongoing Circulation is necessary for nourishment and oxygen to be received; i.e., necessary to continue to exist and thrive.

Frequent use of technology serves like a heart; if it stops for very long your ability to function will be dangerously compromised.

- *Pathway to Technology Number 4*: **Share the wealth—Be a Mentor.** *Learn it, Do it, Teach it*—This epitaph is engraved in the minds of educators. If you really want to learn a concept or skill then do it frequently and teach it often. Not only will this help with retention but it will increase the use of technology among peers as well. No one person can serve as a mentor for a large number of people. If you have a good mentor, then you can model this service to others with the shared expectation that those you mentor will do the same. Mentoring is like donating blood; the donor may feel a little weak after giving, but the recipient receives a gift that increases the circulation of oxygen rich red blood cells—the gift of life.

Key Technological Experiences

Many faculty teaching predominately online courses are experienced with the latest learning technology and offer much regarding its use and value. Traditional classroom instructors know the merit of the face-to-face encounter; the ability to instantly assess from the group adequate understanding versus confusion and boredom or disinterest. Blending online learning with live, interpersonal experiences provides students and faculty the best of both worlds. Individually, chocolate and peanut butter taste good. Combined, the deliciousness of chocolate with the nutritional value of peanut butter provides a unique mix of sweetness and saltiness satisfying to the palate. Blending online teaching with live experiences provides positive outcomes for both the student and teacher.

Blended or Hybrid courses are those that include online and in class activities and encourage independent learning. (Garnham and Kaleta, 2002)—a skill needed for life long learning. Online preparation for class provides the student with the information most important to know and understand before lecture so that the classroom experience can focus on application and other higher cognitive levels of the lecture concepts. Faculty are not only spared precious class time covering basic knowledge, administering quizzes, etc., but instantly maintain an ongoing record of each student's investment in preparing for class and the course—a valuable insight. An exploration of key technologies available and how these tools can be used everyday will illuminate the possibilities.

KEY TECHNOLOGIES AVAILABLE

Course Management Systems [CMS]

Most colleges and universities use a course management system [CMS] to organize and expedite online learning. A CMS is just what it says, a method for faculty to organize and publish a course online. These systems provide excellent opportunities for teaching, learning, and ongoing communication with course enrolled students and are most frequently used by online courses and programs. Traditional colleges and universities are encouraging campus based faculty to use CMS's to help organize and facilitate learning. As with any new technology, time and frequent experience—repetition—are assisting new faculty and faculty new to the CMS to effectively utilize the system. Beware that initially the use of the CMS may seem a bit overwhelming and time-consuming. However, with a good mentor you can quickly overcome your inadequacies and find the time well worth the front-end effort. In fact, teaching and student learning may be negatively affected without the CMS.

WebCT — http://www.webct.com/, *Blackboard* — http://www.blackboard.com/, and *ANGEL [A New Global Environment for Learning]* — http://www.angellearning.com/, are the most commonly purchased course management systems. Another CMS available at no cost is *Moodle* — http://moodle.org/. *Moodle* is especially beneficial if your institution does not possess a CMS. *Moodle* is also useful to build remediation course sites to help prepare your nursing program's graduates for the NCLEX-RN™ exam after graduation. Most purchased packages do not allow graduates to access the CMS since they are no longer officially enrolled students, thus, *Moodle* becomes a great resource in this situation.

Applications Available in Course Management Systems

CMS software packages come with different applications and allow universities to purchase licensing agreements for access and use. "Learning without limits" is the slogan descriptor for *WebCT* and very accurately defines what the CMS does—it is the vehicle of e-learning. A CMS offers multiple resources to assist faculty in course design, more than can be described in this chapter but covered in depth at each CMS website. CMS's serve four primary purposes: 1) *Communication*—Faculty to Student Group, Faculty to Individual Student, and Student to Student;

2) *Learning*—both Guided and Self Directed, 3) *Assessment and Evaluation*—Formative and Summative; and 4) *an Archive of Course Activities and Events* that is easily accessed to supply data for curricular decisions required by accreditation bodies.

Communication Uses

Initially, the CMS is most valued for its course communication capabilities of the course syllabus and policies, course email, events calendar, and the ongoing reporting and recording of student grades, which dismisses the need of double documentation of student scores by hardcopy or spreadsheet file, provides the individual student ongoing progress reports, and expedites the submission of official grade transmissions to the institution's records office with very little effort from faculty. Course information that generally remains constant from one semester to the next can be backed up and stored in a CMS, allowing easy access and copy retrieval to update the next semester the course is taught. Making revisions based on calendar changes and on identified areas for improvement becomes an easy task.

Syllabus—"I lost my syllabus. What is the grading criterion?" How many times do we hear these questions and then spend precious time helping students locate the information. A CMS publishes this information 24/7 anywhere in the world as long as the enrolled student has Internet access.

Course Policies with Hyperlinks to Program and/or University Policies—Students can with the touch of a button see how one policy flows from another and the connectedness. Students maintain easy, electronic access to the rules and can no longer say, "I did not know that was a policy" or "Where is that written?" Students often violate policies that are published in obscure places—like the "University Catalog or Bulletin." These documents are obscure, you ask? To an eighteen year old, a university catalog is like the very fine print on a legal transaction, something you know you should probably read but do not take time to do so. By the way, when was the last time you read your university's catalog? Get the picture.

Another advantage is that the mere process of setting up hyperlinks allows faculty to scrutinize existing policies and confirm that current course, program and university statements do not conflict—a legal safety net for you, your program, and your university.

WARNING: Do not make changes in the course syllabus or policies during the semester unless legal counsel advises the immediate revision.

Course Calendar—The course calendar provides a quick reference for you and the student to view what is to occur from one day to the next throughout the semester, such as lecture topics for the day with a hyperlink to the reading assignment and lecture objectives, assignments due, and events, including student nursing association meetings and other activities. **WARNING**: Do not change the calendar or any part of the course after the first day of class without first consulting all students. Changes in a calendar are inevitable, but students legitimately resent discovering amendments from a surprise calendar revision. In fact, such a change is not fair and can damage the faculty-student relationship. Needed adjustments can be discussed at the beginning of a class and can easily be made in the CMS during this meeting with the LCD Projector illuminating the change on the screen for the students to visualize.

Email—Faculty and students are capable of emailing without a CMS. However, a CMS keeps a copy of each email exchanged during the entire course and stores this information when the course is saved at the end of the semester. As a faculty member, you have evidence of each interaction at your fingertips inside the course, not crowding and jumbling up your university email files. An email icon exists on the entry page for each course and is highlighted when there is unread mail for all course participants—students and faculty.

Discussion Boards—The Discussion Board is a method of exchanging information and ideas among students, faculty, and the entire class if desired. Gone are the days that you are required to explain a difficult concept to one student at a time following lecture. The discussion board allows difficult concepts to be addressed so that every student has the advantage of learning from the exchange. Discussion boards decrease the guilt that you may experience after clarifying a concept for one person but not for others who may be just as confused. Furthermore, the board frees faculty time to answer questions once rather than three, four, or more times and lets students attempt to help each other explain concepts with your supervision. This application is discussed further under learning applications.

Student Performance—Many student questions faculty delight in answering and others we dread to hear. "What are my grades for the semester?" "I can't find my second test score what was it?" A CMS keeps the student informed of every grade in the course when you, the faculty, are ready for the student to retrieve it. Students merely access the "My Grades" icon in the CMS course and determine not only the grade for every assignment, exam, and quiz, but also his/her ongoing average for the course. If a quiz or assignment is submitted within the CMS, the grade is automatically stored in the teacher's grade file as well, eliminating the need to hand record grades. Pencil and paper test grades can also be individually added to the teacher's grade file and then released to students as the teacher desires. Confidentiality no longer is an issue. Each individual student is the only person who can access the "My Grades" data. Unfortunately, complaints about scores remains an ongoing problem, but the CMS at least eliminates a faculty's *seek and find* time.

Another advantage of the teacher's grade file is that it performs like a spreadsheet program. The teacher denotes each graded item and percentage for the course and can command the system to calculate final grades. This information is saved within the course and included in the university's CMS's electronic storage, freeing your filing cabinet for current business.

Utilizing your CMS to enhance course and individual communication is only one benefit of the program. How can CMS's improve the learning experience? How can a CMS drive us from a *teach and tell* experience to a *live, learn, and succeed* dimension?

CMS Teaching and Learning Resources

Multiple applications are available in a CMS. The following are a few of my favorites—"My Picks." You as the faculty are free to use the described applications you find most useful for student learning. Be creative and dare to take risks.

Quizzes

A CMS provides a template for developing and administering tests using multiple choice, true/false, fill-in the blank, and essay questions. The faculty selects the type(s) of question(s) for a test. Once completed, quantitative question tests are automatically graded and stored in the teacher's grade file as well as the "My Grades" application. The time once required to reproduce a test can now be used to create more meaningful, NCLEX-RN like questions to assess and evaluate student and group performance, and to enhance learning. Most of the faculty work-time commitment is developing the test banks and planning. Commanding the type of quiz and method of delivery takes less than five minutes.

   The Assessment and Evaluation Quiz—The assessment and evaluation quiz is very much like the traditional classroom quiz or exam but is available online. The advantage of the CMS quiz is that it can be designed based on the purpose intended. For example, if you want to insure students' preparation for lecture, then release a one time quiz that is scheduled to be taken before class. This quiz often utilizes Bloom's (1956) cognitive levels of knowledge and comprehension of the information the student was required to learn prior to class. Most students desire access to class notes before the lecture but do not want to read or prepare. Many of the CMS's applications can be commanded to release information after identified criteria is achieved by the students, for example, students can gain access to lecture notes or outlines once the quiz designed to assist students in preparing for class is completed. Beware, there are differing opinions regarding allowing student access to lecture notes that needs to first be philosophically addressed and determined as a program.

   Evaluation quizzes can be available for students following the classroom experience using higher levels of Bloom's taxonomy—"application, analysis, synthesis, and evaluation" (Bloom, Engelhart, Furst, Hill, & Krathwohl, 1956, pp. 201-207). The teacher can determine the effectiveness of the class experience based on student outcomes and has the data to determine if a correlation exists between class preparation quiz scores and evaluation scores.

   Online quizzing is an exceptional method of teaching, learning, and evaluating student performance, but limitations exist that discourage the use of these tests for major course exams. Faculty can restrict the test-taking time, which may deter cheating especially if only one minute is allotted per question. However, students can print out copies of the test, which breaches test security. This problem is addressed by many newer programs that disallow printing of a page and/or copying and pasting of information into another file. However, newer computers contain built in cameras that can capture an image of any page accessed. Until this issue is adequately addressed, the security of online testing within the CMS remains questionable.

The Eternal Quiz—A Win-Win Learning Experience—The *eternal quiz* is self-explanatory—the student can take the quiz as many times as he/she wants until the grade desired is achieved. This quiz can actually be devised to accept only the highest grade, or an average of all the individual student's grades within a quiz. Both students and faculty win when the highest achieved score is accepted.

The quiz can be designed numerous ways using the CMS quiz application. Students can access and complete a quiz as many times as desired but during a prescribed timeframe during the course ranging from days to months. A random selection of questions from a bank will test the students' abilities covering multiple concepts, thus deterring memorization of a small sample of questions. The teacher can command the system to release the test score and to identify which questions were missed but deny release of the correct answer and/or rationale—thus requiring students to return to the literature to find answers. If higher order questions are included, it is not unusual for students to take the quiz 10-12 times before achieving a 100%.

Ideally, these quizzes cover critical information from the NCSBN's Nursing Activities Study, JCAHO's Sentinel Events and Patient Safety Goals, and nursing and pharmacological basics. Students admit feeling empowered by eternal quizzes—because the repetition ingrains important concepts into their brains and they find using this data assists in clinical decision making in class case studies and the clinical setting.

Gaming

What words come to mind when you think of being tested—work, terror? Does the phrase, "Get out a sheet of paper," implying a pop test is about to occur, cause an undesirable psychological and physiological reaction? What is your response to the word "play" or "game?" Remember what students feel when testing occurs—anxiety and fear. But what if we provided gaming experiences for student learning? The term "game" indicates fun may actually be an outcome of the experience. Why not provide learning encounters that are as addictive as computer games? What could be better than learning while playing?

Learning can be fun when faculty download game templates from their

CMS website and develop activities for students to gain facts about important concepts. Gaming is becoming a popular learning application to meet the computer literate generation's needs. These students teethed on computers and game programs, making the use of such more appealing. Many CMS's contain packages that include interactive games that can be adapted to nursing education. Audio flash cards, video animations, and virtual environments, are a few examples. Critical thinking exercises are available as well. But for the teacher who cringes at the word "fun," requirements for students to learn without enjoyment still exists, but hopefully this does not describe you.

The Discussion Board as a Learning Tool—Do you ever find yourself conducting Google searches that produce rich data from incredibly reliable sources but neglecting to even scan the information because of a lack of time? Do you review your nursing text chapter only to find the most critical information for a lecture missing or under-emphasized? Try using the discussion board to post hyperlinks to specific websites and to entice students to access the sites by guaranteeing a 100% quiz score if they select, read, and post on the discussion board 1) a synopsis of one of the listed articles, 2) cite the reference, 3) identify how the article effects nursing practice, and 4) describe their personal reactions. This experience generally results in students who come to class with questions and opinions that generate dynamic interactions in the classroom. Your workload is decreased but the student outcomes are increased.

Online Assignments—The Paperless Classroom—Lost assignments via student or faculty, problems encountered when a student's assignment needs to be double graded, the laborious lugging of student papers to grade—how can these issues be resolved in a snap? A paperless course eliminates each of these problems and reduces the use of paper, ink, and in many cases, faculty time. The CMS will contain an Assignment Application that can be utilized for almost any course requirement. Faculty can create templates of assignments, include directions, and then publish via the CMS course. Students can download the template, complete the requirement, and resubmit without leaving their computers. Faculty can command the system to provide an automatic email to each student confirming the assignment was received. A CMS records the exact date and time the assignment was submitted and allows faculty to download each individual's assignment or expedite the download of all student work simultaneously by using the *WinZip* program — http://www.winzip.com/. Grading word processed documents versus handwritten work is easy on the eyes, but more importantly, exercises students' computer skills.

One primary limitation to online grading is that it limits faculty without laptop computers to grade at stationary, desk top computers. Laptops with wireless abilities can easily access and upload assignments from an available wireless network, but laptops without wireless capabilities must be directly connected to an Internet server to upload and return graded work via the CMS. Uploaded assignments are saved to the faculty's computer so that actual grading activities do not require Internet access.

Once an assignment is evaluated by faculty, the document is uploaded into the course to return to the student, which prompts a comment section for qualitative feedback and a box to document the student's score. Each student's outcome is automatically recorded in the CMS grade file and the "My Grades" record.

Surveys —"I really wish I knew the students' perception regarding..." This question frequently enters teachers' minds, but the time and effort consumed by developing, copying, administering, and tabulating the results of a survey deter gathering ongoing input from students regarding the learning experience. We often ask students in person about the event and they eagerly tell us what we long to hear, "Oh, it was great! I loved it!" a self-protective response for the person being evaluated and music to the ears of the evaluator. But, is the data accurate and beneficial to use for improvements?

The survey application of a CMS allows questions to be addressed anonymously, with limited faculty effort and eliminates the disturbance of class time to gather the data. Questions debated among team teaching faculty regarding student preferences are resolved by a quick, online survey that requires less than two to three minutes to develop and publish. Team decisions are then based on feedback from the entire student group.

The Survey application of both the *Respondus*® software package and the CMS is a most valuable method of obtaining student input. The application can be used for formative and summative evaluation thus decreasing costs of paper, copying, recording qualitative comments into a word processing file to reduce student identification of handwritten comments and tabulation of quantifiable outcomes. Students can complete the survey on their own time, which results in more qualitative comments and recommendations. Individual faculty can use the survey to determine student perceptions of teaching performance throughout the semester, to answer questions emerging from team-taught faculty that benefit from student input, and to evaluate a learning experience, course, and program of study.

Surveys can also give faculty insight to a student group's learning. Years of using a variety of teaching methods to cover cultural aspects of nursing yielded less than desirable results. One year, I decided that all the work was not worth the effort and simply utilized a campus-wide "World Day" event to expose students to diverse populations, cultures, and such. Students were given detailed instructions of how to initiate encounters, topics to discuss, etc., with individuals from cultures different from their own. Students received a 100% quiz grade by attending the event and completing a three question anonymous survey. The survey application protects anonymity of the reporter but allows faculty to determine who completed the survey and who did not. Students were not graded on what they said, just merely the completion of the requirement. Here are only a few of the comments retrieved:

> "At first I was a little uncomfortable, because I felt like I was there for the wrong reason. However, after I loosened up, and danced and really got involved in their dance, and music, I felt more comfortable. I stopped thinking of it like a class project and more of just getting to know some new interesting people who were very open and caring...I have a lot more I would like to talk to them about then I had an opportunity to at the event."

> "I learned a lot about Argentina from a couple I talked to. It was information I probably could not have gotten from a text or lecture. I really enjoyed that part."

> "I felt ashamed that I had not spent more time getting to know people from other cultures and that I didn't really know how to relate in a lot of ways. I felt bad for complaining about having to come because I had such a good time."

> "Sometimes people from other cultures accuse our culture for leaving them out or being partial to one side over the other. But as I looked around, I saw what they were saying, but I also saw they did the same thing too. So whether we want to admit it or not, every one is so similar it's funny."

> "In all honesty, its not that I really learned a lot about another culture, but I became aware that these different cultures that are present in our society have specific needs that should be met. I have become more aware of the

different cultures that I am in contact with everyday. I am close friends with a guy from Portugal....After this event, I decided just to interview him and really understand how he feels in the society. It is amazing how thankful and excited he is to be here. His testimony is unbelievable and truly shows how many cultures that are in the United States have been burdened with many trials. This event made me want to really understand where they are coming from and the trials they have experienced. Many times we are so comfortable where we are, we forget that our next door neighbor is hurting and is in need."

"I think I learned about myself.... I learned that I am fortunate, and that given the chance, anyone can become a friend."

"I learned that I personally had some distorted views of other cultures, but that by spending time with others who are different from us we can better ourselves and our view of the world (and have a really good time)."

"...the world is a lot broader place than you think about it being and most people are very willing to share their experiences with you if you only ask."

"I learned from the people that I talked to that while we have differences, we also have many of the same goals in life: family, work and security. A lot of us are not as different as we think."

"Truly, after talking to someone for about 45 minutes all I really got from this person was the difference in food. He was talking about how much cheese and mayonnaise there was in the United States."

Many themes emerged from the survey, but most impressive was the stirring of the intrinsic drive to learn more from others. Good learning experiences need not be burdensome to the faculty or students. A survey frees students to state their true thoughts and feelings. The online survey provides insights to the learning experience with legitimate findings.

My Pages

A CMS includes not only a multitude of directed applications, but also pages the faculty can personalize and develop to assist students in achieving course objectives. A Resource page that includes some of the most valuable and reliable resource sites for students is beneficial in directing students to differentiate legitimate versus questionable Internet sites and sources. The following are only a few hyperlinks that assist nursing students in obtaining valid and reliable data.

Resources—Critical Resources Sites for Nursing Education
- **American Nurses' Association's Nursing World:**
  http://www.nursingworld.org/
- **Center for Disease Control [CDC]** http://www.cdc.gov/
- **Joint Commission on the Accreditation of Healthcare Organizations**
  - http://www.jcaho.org/
  - Patient Safety: http://www.jcipatientsafety.org/
  - Sentinel Events:
    http://www.jcipatientsafety.org/show.asp?durki=9336
- **National Council for the State Board of Nursing:**
  - http://www.ncsbn.org/
  - Learning Extension: http://www.learningext.com/
- **National Institutes of Health:** http://www.nih.gov/

Assessment and Evaluation Abilities of the CMS

A CMS is the easiest way to expedite the continuous quality improvement process. Formative and summative assessment, improvement/learning, and evaluation can be studied on multiple levels—individual student, course, faculty, clinical experience, and program. You can download your program's instruments to access and store the outcomes of each survey. These outcomes can be used to drive improvement efforts at all levels and serve as data to make curricular decisions—an invaluable resource for accreditation visits.

Archives and Storage
A CMS allows faculty to save and store each course taught. Easy access to past courses is extremely beneficial to provide information for continuous quality improvement efforts and accreditation bodies.
- *Pathway to Technology Number 5*: **Use your institution's course management system to enhance learning and to save yourself time.**

Programs Beyond the CMS

Respondus® — A Teacher's Best Friend http://www.respondus.com/

One beneficial software package is *Respondus®*, a test development and bank that stores questions from all your courses. *Respondus®* allows you to maintain ongoing test bank files that can be easily downloaded into any course. With a simple click beside a question in a test bank, the teacher can select which questions to include and exclude in each exam. The primary advantage to *Respondus®* is that you can access the test bank without resurrecting a CMS archived course, i.e., access questions that may be used in other courses or that can serve as remediation activities for graduates preparing for NCLEX-RN™ . Revision and electronic storage of test items as well as survey questions without retyping or copying and pasting is *Respondus'®* greatest asset. Surveys and tests can easily upload directly into the CMS for online and hardcopy applications.

Respondus® not only serves as a teacher's archive of test questions, but also includes additional resources such as *Respondus® Testbank Network* and *StudyMate*

The *Respondus®* Test Bank Network provides online access to downloadable test banks from identified authors and publishers. For details see the website. Unfortunately, there are few nursing texts to date that offer testbanks in Respondus®, but hopefully this will quickly change as faculty recognize the value of directly downloading a testbank into a Respondus® file and request this service from publishers.

StudyMate 1.1 is an innovative application that provides templates for faculty to develop and download learning games for students. *StudyMate* is available at the *Respondus®* homepage.

The Infamous PowerPoint® by Microsoft® — Boring versus Invigorating

Imagine sitting in a conference after lunch holding a hardcopy of a *PowerPoint®* presentation. The lights are lowered, the screen illuminates, and there, before your very eyes is the exact same information in your possession only larger. The speaker begins and you find yourself being lullabyed into a deep sleep. You can read. Why go to the presentation? The teacher is what brings out the power in *PowerPoint®*. Technology is the vehicle, but the real experience is developed and executed by the faculty — you. Why do we wonder when students fall prey to Mr. Sandman when we give lectures that act as non-pharmaceutical sleep agents?

How do we emphasize the power in *PowerPoint®*? The organization and presentation of the content is crucial. Long, wordy slides are deadly. Converting lecture material into a show is invigorating. Do not underestimate the value of theater and humor. A good performance keeps the participants awake, interested, and eager to experience what will happen next. The content needs to come alive through the presentation of the material. Just as when they watch a good movie, the students should laugh, cry, and become enraged. We want them to experience and learn. *PowerPoint®* presentations are not required for good teaching but can certainly enhance the learning experience if used wisely.

Transforming Lecture into Theater

Images —Add images to your slides. Pictures are easy to find using search engines such as *Google Image* and *Yahoo Image*. These engines provide both graphic photos of diseases, illustrations of anatomy, physiology, and pathophysiology, and also funny cartoons that may emphasize a point or absurdity. When using an image, be certain to cite the reference on the slideshow presentation with the graphic. Many companies that release images on the Internet allow educators to use the work without official written consent, but it is safest to request first. If the document states that it cannot be reproduced, then find another image or ask the author for special permission.

Sounds —I believe in stimulating as many senses as possible during lecture. If I could bottle the smell of flatulence, I would release it in the air when discussing disease processes, foods, etc., that produce gas as a symptom. I have yet to master how to reproduce olfactory stimuli in class without humiliating myself but find that auditory stimuli are easy to access and include in *PowerPoint®* presentations. Numerous free sound bytes exist that can be downloaded for free and placed in the presentation at the most appropriate moments. For example, when discussing Angiotensin Converting Enzyme antihypertensive drugs, I click on the sound wave included on the slide that produces a dry cough. I click and re-click this sound—which takes no longer than five seconds—until the class realizes something is really important about this cough, that a dry cough is a common side effect of the drug that often causes patients to discontinue treatment.

Learners smile when they see the little sound horn icon on the slide knowing that something is about to occur that is either humorous, informative, or both. When I address a major complication, I click on Tom Hank's voice from Apollo 13 stating, "Houston, we have a problem!" Students quickly learn that this means the patient's situation is serious and could be life threatening if not addressed immediately. Most sound bytes last less than two seconds in reality but have lasting learning effects.

Free Sound Byte Sources:
- *Wav Source:* http://www.wavsource.com/
- *Partners in Rhyme:*
  http://www.partnersinrhyme.com/pir/PIRsfx.html
- *Tintagel's Free Sound Files:*
  http://freesoundfiles.tintagel.net/Audio/

Movies —Experience Hollywood; make a movie! Develop a short film to play before class—while students are filing in—that focuses on major concepts in a fun and lively way. Include legally purchased music and images. Include students in the movie-making learning process to improve computer competency skills and to assist in the development of creative videos for teaching/learning assignments that can be archived and used by future students, faculty, and the community. Be certain to have some fun in the process.

Movie Software
- Microsoft® Windows® Moviemaker
- Apple—iLife—iMovie—My educator friends experienced with both the Windows Moviemaker and Apple iMovie prefer iMovie to Moviemaker primarily because of the ease of use.

Games

Virtual Classroom
Elluminate is software that provides the opportunity for audio/video streaming—live and/or recorded classroom experiences, web conferencing, instant messaging, and more. *Elluminate* is universally accessible

through an Internet connection regardless of the institution's or individual student's operating system, Windows or Mac, and can function even with 28.8 dial-up connection—especially useful to rural students without cable or satellite capabilities.

Elluminate offers numerous possibilities for online and blended class experiences—live or recorded lecture for students who require repetition to re-experience the class, breakout rooms (the ability to break the student population into small groups in which only the instructor and people in the session can visualize and hear the conversation), and group discussions. The professor can switch between breakout rooms and provide assistance, interject advice, or review progress without disturbing the process. Elluminate is especially beneficial during testing since students can be easily placed into breakout rooms for faculty observation, thus reducing cheating.

- *__Pathway to Technology Number 6:__* **Technology is only as good as its contents.** If the concepts covered are insufficient, disorganized, overloaded, and/or poorly delivered the outcomes will suffer. Remember, it is the teacher's responsibility to construct the course and learning experience—technology is the vehicle of delivery.

Conclusion

Chickering and Gamson describe seven principles for good practice in higher education to include 1) ongoing contact between students and faculty, 2) student exchange and cooperation, 3) active learning, 4) prompt feedback from faculty, 5) an emphasis regarding time on task, 6) communication of high expectations, and, 7) respect for diverse talent and ways of learning. Well designed courses utilizing technology as a vehicle of learning is the method by which each of these seven principles can be achieved. http://honolulu.hawaii.edu/intranet/committees/FacDevCom/guidebk/teachtip/7princip.htm

Technology is like medicine—ever-changing. What is current today is ancient tomorrow. Strive to ride the waves of change. Be the one to venture down the pathway to learning that is technologically driven. Avoid negative teachers who want the environment to remain constant, because it will not. Surround yourself with innovators, shakers and movers—and become one.

Important concepts

- **A good rapport and working relationship with your institution's technology department is vital to success.**

- **Search for a mentor and become his/her Cling-On.**

- **Utilize and value technologically savvy faculty.**

- **Use your institution's CMS to the fullest extent—the extra planning time on the front end is worth the investment.**

- **Remember, technology is only as good as its contents and designed learning experiences.**

- **Dare to take technological risks.**

Acknowledgements

To my mentor, Dr. Robert Clougherty, who continuously empowers me to use technology beyond my comfort to promote student learning.

References

American Nurses' Association's Nursing World. Retrieved June 7, 2005 from *http://www.nursingworld.org/*

A New Global Environment for Learning [ANGEL]. Retrieved October 30, 2005 from *http://www.angellearning.com/*

Banta, T. (1995). This one's for students. *Assessment Update*. 7, 3, 3 & 13.

Bloom, B., Engelhart, M., Furst, E., and Krathwohl, D. (1956). Taxonomy of educational objectives: The classification of educational goals. New York: David McKay Company, Inc.

Center for Disease Control. Retrieved May 31, 2005 from http://www.cdc.gov/

Chickering and Gamon. TBA http://honolulu.hawaii.edu/intranet/committees/FacDevCom/guidebk/teachtip/7princip.htm

Elluminate. Retrieved June 11, 2005 from http://www.elluminate.com/

Garnham, C. and Kaleta, R. (2002). Introduction to hybrid courses. *Teaching with Technology Today*, 8, 6. Retrieved June 14, 2004 from http://www.uwsa.edu/ ttt/articles/garnham.htm

iMovie by Apple. Retrieved June 11, 2005

Joint Commission on Accreditation of Healthcare Organizations. Retrieved May 31, 2005 from http://www.jcaho.org/

Movie Maker by Microsoft. Retrieved June 14, 2005

National Council of State Boards of Nursing. Retrieved May 31, 2005 from
  http://www.ncsbn.org/

National Institute of Health. Retrieved May 31, 2005 from http://www.nih.gov/

Office PowerPoint by Microsoft. Retrieved June 7, 2005

Partners in Rhyme. Retrieved June 7, 2005 from
  http://www.partnersinrhyme.com/pir/PIRsfx.html

Respondus®. Retrieved May 31, 2005 from http://www.respondus.com/

Tintagel's Free Sound Files. Retrieved June 7, 2005 from
  http://freesoundfiles.tintagel.net/Audio/

Wav Source. Retrieved June 7, 2005 from http://www.wavsource.com/

WebCT. Retrieved May 31, 2005 from http://www.webct.com/

WinZip. Retrieved June 7, 2005 from http://www.winzip.com/

Chapter 8

THE PATH TO KEEPING CLINICAL ASSIGNMENTS REAL

"They may forget what you said, but they will never forget how you made them feel."
Carl W. Buechner

Have you ever looked at your new clinical group and thought to yourself, "Who did this to me?" Talk about a challenge! Clinical Teaching is a verb. *It is not supervision, it is guidance. It is something that you do, not something that you let happen and then evaluate.* Where do we start? We start with the same place we started with our class. Establishing relationships is path number 1 in any challenge. Let them know that you have been in their shoes and you are there to help them. Start with the W's that we have discussed in Chapter 3.

Ask the learner how you can help them be successful. This is a technique that is so vitally important that we don't use it frequently enough.

Many clinical faculty believe that the student has to develop a 21 page nursing care plan on their patient before they can attend clinical. This means that the faculty has to go to the hospital agency the day before, even if it is on Sunday, their day off, to determine which patient the student will care for. The student then stays up all night completing the care plan, comes to clinical the next day exhausted and we want to know why they don't think! If this is not stressful enough, their patient may have died or been discharged. Now the student is angry because they know that their work will not "count" because they have no patient.

Have we ever stopped to think that the new graduate does not complete this lengthy care plan before they come to work? They wait until they get to work and assess their patient before planning their day. *We need to give the students the tools to work in the real world.* We can do this from the first day by teaching them quick, real-time assessment skills and then providing them a pre-conference time to help them analyze their assessment and plan the care that they can complete this day. We need to emphasize how they can help their patients survive this day in the hospital. Research has shown us that we should have an advocate when we are hospitalized. There is such a tremendous nursing shortage that hospitals are not always the safest place to be. Help them plan safety for their patients for this clinical day. Pre-conference is a vital part of clinical teaching. A space must be found to have it and reference books will be needed. We can assign students to bring certain books. For example, one can bring a laboratory manual, one a drug handbook, one a nursing book, or other resource. This way they have the tools that they need for pre-conference. It is also important that they have a copy of the care plan or concept map that the agency uses. This way they can plan *on the spot*.

This brings us to another discussion, hospital or other agency expectations. Who is going to do the beds and baths while the students are in pre-conference? Many hospitals give their nursing assistant staff the day off if the students are coming. That means that there is no one else to give the patients baths and change their bed linen. We have to revisit this expectation of our students. How do they have time to learn if they are busy with the same tasks every time they go into the hospital? They don't. We need to establish relationships with the staff as well. We need them and they need us. We cannot allow them to expect that students will always be available to do beds and baths.

Every department of nursing has an "agency agreement" with the hospitals and other agencies that they use for clinical experience. It is typically kept in the department head's office. Take a look at that written agreement, because as faculty, you are legally responsible for abiding by this agreement. Every one of these agreements says that the department of nursing is responsible for the student learning. It does not say that every student is responsible for doing the beds and baths for the agencies' patients. But, you say the agencies demand that this expectation continue! We have to plan with the agency staff the semester before we plan to change this expectation, letting the agencies know what the learners will be doing. They want and need competent and capable new graduates. They do not want to give their staff the day off and then the instructor to come in and say, "Oh, by the way, we're not going to do the beds and baths today". *Planning ahead is a beautiful thing! It allows everyone to have a paradigm shift without a crisis.*

Clinical faculty are often the ones "dragging their feet" with this change. They will use words like, "The bath is the best time to do an assessment." Well, the bath is a good time to do an assessment, but we cannot be in the position of teaching the new student that they only way that they can do an assessment is to give a bath. In the real world they do not have the luxury of this much time.

We believe that we, as nursing faculty, may have contributed to the nursing shortage with some of our outdated teaching methods. Many new graduates are scared to death to go to their first job because they do not have a care plan on all their patients. They do not know how to do a quick assessment. They have way too much to do in the short time that they have with the clients and they grow disillusioned. I don't know where they go in your part of the world, but in ours, they quit nursing and start selling real estate. *We have to give them tools to work with in today's environment.* We need to help them learn to feel good about the things that they get done, not bad about the things they did not get done. The only way that we know how to do this is to help them learn how to prioritize. Let them learn using experiential learning so that they can think on their feet.

Some of our new nurses worry that they cannot make life-saving decisions because they do not have the plan or the chart in their hands. They have to be confident in answering the client's light and knowing what action to take if the client is short of breath, having crushing chest pain or is bleeding out of the IV.

Many nursing care plans are utilized by faculty as documentation for a clinical grade or proof that they have prepared for their clinical assignment. We all know that many students copy care plans from care plan books. This does not mean that they have done any type of critical thinking about a patient. A nursing care plan says what a student can do, it does not say what a student will do. There is a world of difference. This is where clinical evaluation comes in.

While following this path, it is also imperative to review the role model behaviors necessary in the clinical setting. Wiseman (1994) asserts, "In nursing education, the faculty member serves as the primary role-model initiating the student into the profession". The role model behaviors identified in Wiseman's study has been organized around the acronym "**TIP**".

TIP	
T	Technical Know-How Thinking (Critical)
I	Interpersonal Effectiveness
P	Professional Role Behaviors

It goes without saying that faculty who role mode **"TIP"** are very effective with students. These are the faculty that truly inspire optimal growth and development in their students.

To keep clinical assignments real, then successive assignments should build on each student's progress. "A sequence of experiences that has both continuity and connection is important." (Fothergill-Bourbonnais & Higuchi, 1995, p. 40) The design of successive assignments should build on each student's progress. These are outlined in **"TRACKS"**. This acronym has been adapted from this research. Always remember that faculty "**tracks**" the progress of students throughout the learning experience.

TRACKS	
T	Technical skill development
R	Responsiveness to an increasing number of client variables
A	Ability to organize and manage a complex assignment Achieve independence in making decisions and clinical judgments
C	Complex care demands are able to be managed
K	Knowledge to be able to recognize typical, then atypical patterns of response
S	Safety

The clinical instructor must consider the individual abilities of the students in the clinical group, and select learning opportunities accordingly. The instructor must tailor assignments to allow each student to progress steadily toward the final goal. We always like to share with our students the rationale for making specific assignments so the student could focus on the priority learning opportunity. As the students mature and develop, they may request specific clinical experiences. These requests need to be honored if it is possible. These requests are also other indicators that the student is following the *"path of learning with ownership!"* Each of these paths are like building blocks and are all connected.

Chapter 9

THE PATH TO REAL CLINICAL EVALUATION

"The secret of joy in work is contained in one word - excellence.
To know how to do something well is to enjoy it."
Pearl S. Buck

There is more time and consternation spent on clinical evaluation tools than most nursing faculty have to give to this task. Many departments have "global" clinical evaluation tools that support nebulous objectives. Then when they go to the department head and dean to say that a student has a failing clinical grade, they are "not supported" with the clinical failure because they "do not have proper documentation". This error happens so often that clinical faculty get to the point that they refuse to give a student a clinical failure because they know that they may not be supported.

One size does not fit all. It is very hard to utilize the same tool for every course because the course objectives are so varied. They should be varied. That's the reason we have different courses.

The clinical evaluation tool is one of the most important pieces of paper in a course. It should candidly spell out student expectations. The students should have this evaluation tool in their hands before they ever enter the hospital agency the first time. This is called due process. This means the nursing faculty have to agree on the expectations of clinical for each course. Many nursing programs try to utilize the exact same tool for every single course. If we customize the evaluation tools to the course objectives, we will have a stronger program with more direction.

Where do the objectives that should be spelled out on the clinical evaluation tool come from? First the program objectives should be carried through in the clinical objectives. These program objectives should originate with the objectives of the University or College. At a minimum, the nursing standards as documented through research by the National Council of State Boards of Nursing (NCSBN) must be considered as objectives. There are usually less than 200 of these minimum standards that come from the "RN Practice Analysis" that is completed every three years to supply the framework for the NCLEX-RN™ examination. These minimum standards should be spelled out in course and clinical objectives, content preparation, course examinations and clinical evaluations.

Clinical evaluation is about the learner being safe and effective as a practitioner. It is not about how well the learner can write a care plan. The Board of Nursing in each state contracts with the NCSBN as they are evaluating the safety of care by the new graduate. The agencies that hire our new graduates want to know if they are safe. How can we determine their safety if we do not hold them accountable for the minimum standard of nursing? For example, one of the most important and current standards is that the student demonstrates that they can administer medication utilizing the 5 rights of medication administration. This standard should be on every course and clinical evaluation tool. Another standard example is that the student utilize infection control standards. This also is a concept that should be an objective on every clinical evaluation tool.

We can utilize nursing research conducted by the NCSBN to help us develop our minimum clinical tool. Now we have a tool that can be supported. For example, did they demonstrate the use of the 5 rights of medication administration? The answer is often yes or no. If no, the faculty documents how they did not perform utilizing this minimum standard. There now is no question of support. The did it or they didn't and the personal observations by an educational observer are in evidence.

One cannot stop with an observation if the student fails to meet the objective. To follow due process, the student must be counseled that they did not meet the objective, how to meet it and the consequences if they do not meet it the next time. All of this procedure must be in writing with the student's signature that they have been counseled. Appropriate "Due Process" keeps clinical faculty within their scope of practice and out of courtrooms. Some students believe that they only way that they can be heard is to sue. Here is where we go back to path number 1. Students rarely sue nursing faculty that they like. *Relationship, relationship, relationship is the key.*

There are probably more institutions that grade with a pass/fail in clinical than using a sliding scale that gives a grade of A, B, C, D, F. Most pass/fail tools are easier to use; however, faculty utilizing this kind of form tend to add a third "needs improvement" column. Accountability often falls by the wayside with this third column. Faculty will provide the student in every semester with evaluations that say "needs for improvement".

The student then graduates, fails the NCLEX-RN™ and the faculty says, "I knew they would never pass." Where is the faculty accountability in this evaluation system? If a "needs improvement" column must be added, at least consider advising the student that this improvement must be evident before the end of the semester when the third column goes away and there is only the pass/fail column left.

How do we give a clinical grade if we have no nursing care plan, drug cards, concept maps, etc., that can be graded for evidence? What can take the place of these written tools? The answer is simple. There is NO written work that should be graded. The student is graded on their clinical performance alone. The written work is not evidence of the execution of the nursing care that the student will do: it may be evidence of how well they can copy from a nursing care plan book.

There are at least a couple of ways to make sure that the learner actually is accountable for the client's nursing care. The first is to make certain that the learner has the opportunity to meet the course objectives through their clinical experiences. This can be a hard task. Sometimes we are amazed at how well students hide! We have to provide them with a challenge and give them the guidance and opportunity to meet the clinical objectives. Some people call this "setting up". We believe we set ourselves and the safety of our clients up when we allow the student to hide and when we refuse to assign them to the difficult patients. This is called aiding and abetting.

Some faculty believe that if they assign a "poor student" to a sick patient that this assignment will take all of the faculty time. They are right! You have to watch a "poor" student, document their behavior and help them with the tough decision making. Now, you say, "But this is not fair to the smart students." You know, the smart student will come and get you if they need you. You cannot always depend on the poor student to make that decision. That is one of the definitions of "poor".

Look at an example of a clinical assignment/evaluation tool for an early course in nursing at Level 1.

SAMPLE CLINICAL ASSIGNMENT/EVALUATION TOOL	
Meet the dress code and professional behavior outlined by the university and the hospital agency **Determine if vital signs are abnormal** **Assess peripheral pulses**	
1	Apply principles of infection control
2	Verify identity of the client
3	Assess client's discomfort or pain
4	Protect client from injury
5	Identify changes in respiratory status
6	Document client care
7	Notify others of client's change in status

This tool can be used the first week the student is in clinical. Let's discuss each of these starting with "meet dress code." Faculty do not want the student to show up with green hair, rings in their noses, wearing jeans and showing their belly skin. Learners should be apprised of the professional dress code and conduct before they even know where to park their car at the clinical agency. This comes under one of the "W's" that we discussed in an earlier chapter, simplified as *What to Wear*. It's at the top of the list and encompasses not showing up under the influence of drugs, alcohol etc. If the learner fails to meet this objective, we believe they should never have the opportunity to take the first vital sign. If they show up in an unacceptable dress or inebriated and we allow them to begin nursing care on the client, we have given them permission to do this over and over again. We must evaluate the objectives on day one. Of course, they have to have a learning curve, but how they show up on the clinical unit is not a part of a learning curve. It is a clear decision on their part of their intention of meeting the first objective. This objective should be made very clear to the learner very early.

The second objective, determine if vital signs are abnormal, should be explained to the learner. We want them to know that they are responsible for taking the vital signs themselves and at this point in their learning cycle, may not depend on someone else's reading. This means that in the nursing department lab, prior to assignment to the clinical agency, they will have been taught:

- How to approach the client: unconscious, asleep, bandaged, up in chair, withdrawn etc.

- How to evaluate the cuff size and type to use, for example do not use a pediatric cuff on a 300 pound person as it may cut their arm. The client taking coumadin may not be able to tolerate a "hard cuff" because of bruising.

- How to listen to all five Korotkoff blood pressure sounds, as in, be sure the pulse is obliterated by the cuff before they quit pumping the cuff up. They may only measure the lower 2 sounds and totally miss the high sounds.

- How to measure the pulse, yes, they will need some type of watch with a "second hand".

- How to count respirations.

- Know what "normals" are for all 3 of these vital signs. If they do not know normal ranges they cannot determine if they are abnormal.

- How to find and count peripheral pulses and what the name of the pulses are called.

We are now to number one of our list of urgent actions: apply principles of infection control. The bottom line here is that we do not want them taking the client's vital signs if they have not washed their hands. Yes, this means an infection control, hand washing lab before going to the clinical agency.

Number 2 We do not want them taking vital signs of the client if they do not know who the clients is. They must know how to accurately get the identity of the client. (10 minutes in the lab).

Number 3 Ask the client about any pain they are having or if taking the vital sign causes pain. (Lab on how to look at the face and other clues for pain evaluation).

Number 4 Do not stand the patient up for "standing blood pressures" if they are unconscious! Keep the side rails up if needed. Note if fall protocol is posted. (Short lab on fall protocol-another 10 minutes).

Number 5 If they are not breathing, this is not the time to try to hear Korotkoff signs before calling for help!

Number 6 Document. This means that the learner should have seen a flow sheet that the agency uses for documentation prior to their first time in the agency. This lab will take longer than 10 minutes because they have to know how to chart it and how to read the chart if they are adding to a flow sheet.

Number 7 Here is where clinical reasoning takes place. The learner has met all of the other objectives and completed the tasks. Here is the most important part. What are they going to do with the information that they have gathered? Will they dutifully put it on the flow sheet even if it is 220/120? Will they look at the last time it was taken and note that it is elevated? Even if it is not elevated from the last reading, will the clinical reasoning tell them they need to notify someone that the BP medication may not yet be working?

We have to start teaching and modeling clinical reasoning early. DAY ONE. If we do not, they just don't get it.

This complete assignment sheet gives direction to the lab coordinator of where to start in lab as this begins to set the values for the learner. If we start into our first course talking about Florence Nightingale and the Crimean war and how to give a bath and make a bed, we are setting old values. Virtual reality is the name of the game!

Take a close look at this tool again. If you simply draw a vertical column down at the right margin of the page beside all of these objectives you can now have a pass/fail column. Did they dress appropriately and come sober or not? Did they wash their hands or not? Did they notify others of client's change in status? There is no reason for a "needs improvement" column here unless they need to better wash their hands which should have been evaluated in the lab. Just because they wash their hands "right" in lab while you are watching, does not mean they will do the same at the hospital agency. We want to catch them doing something right, but remember, if you see a mistake and do not stop them right then, you are giving them permission to do it over and over again.

This is quite a step by step approach for the opportunity for the learner to meet 10 clinical objectives. Remember there are not that many minimum standards that the learner has to meet to be "safe". We have discussed 10 of them that you have taught, practiced and evaluated within 2 weeks. During the next 2 weeks, there are other minimum standards that need to be taught, practiced and evaluated. Obviously the same clinical assignment and evaluation tools are not used every week, much less in every course. Many faculty say that they do not have time to teach everything, but they do if they have a minimum (revised) focus.

Another key component to this path is providing feedback to the learner that will be informational as well as positively assist in professional growth and development. In our classroom, we use principles of accelerated learning to assist with memory and understanding of difficult nursing concepts. In the clinical area, we use principles of motivational feedback to accelerate professional growth.

As we work with nursing faculty and students, we routinely hear major concerns from new faculty regarding how to motivate students and how to provide them with feedback that will facilitate growth. The situation referred to earlier as being aiding and abetting the "poor students" must STOP now! The next time you assist in this process of allowing a weak student to progress throughout the nursing curriculum just remember he / she could be providing nursing care to you, a family member or a friend.

To prevent this from occurring, motivate by getting the attention of the "EAR". This is a very simple acronym, but these factors are so very powerful!

EAR	
E	Expectations
A	Accountability
R	Reinforcement (Feedback)

"EAR" is universal. They work because they focus on changing behavior! What consistently creates high performance? Let's review each of these factors and find out!

EXPECTATIONS:

People have more positive **expectations** with firstborns. They are going to be the president of the senior class, the all-star-quarterback, etc. Whatever they do they are EXPECTED to succeed.

ACCOUNTABILITY:

Firstborns are given more responsibility and **accountability** at an earlier age. They are asked to look after their sibling. They are responsible and accountable to handle money, the cell phone, directions on how to get to a destination, and what to purchase.

REINFORCEMENT (FEEDBACK):

Firstborns get more **reinforcement** (feedback). They get more attention from family and friends. Parents spend more time with the firstborn than the other children for obvious reasons. I have never known a mother to reprimand a toddler when they were learning to walk. During the learning process we clap, kiss them, and encourage the child to continue!

This is exciting because we have identified three distinct factors that tend to make firstborns better than average achievers. We have had great outcomes from applying these factors to nursing students in the classroom during lecture, in the clinical area, as well as during workshops. Prior to beginning a program or starting with a new clinical group, I always begin with the famous quote by Henry Ford: *"Whether you think you can or you can't, you are right!"* We even state this prior to handing out the evaluation tool, so that I can establish the first essential condition for success and that is creating **"Positive Expectations."**

During weekly sessions with students, they are assisted with the development of meaningful but real learning targets (based on the clinical evaluation tool), based on short-range and long-range goals, so they can achieve success. I hold them **accountable** for being partners in this learning and evaluating process. There is no room for excuses. They have had guidance with this process because novices have no idea what is realistic to achieve at different levels of development. Much of what we do is coaching the clinical group to success. Isn't that what education is all about, **"Bringing Out the Best in Others"**?

Accountability is good, but blame is bad! The Army does a great job in making people accountable without playing the blame game. They teach individuals to take responsibility for both their actions and the failure to act. Unfortunately, by the time most people reach adulthood, they have picked up certain habits such as avoiding responsibility and not facing facts. That is why the army and other military services are so tough during basic training. It takes strong discipline to break bad habits! The army reinforces this retraining by conducting "AARs", that is, *after action review*. Four simple questions are asked:

1. What was supposed to happen?

2. What actually happened?

3. What accounts for any differences?

4. What can be learned?

There is no note-taking. Nothing goes in the personal file. Reviews are simple and straightforward. No blaming — these are learning opportunities. *We must remember there is a time to teach and a time to evaluate!* The first part of clinical is not a time to evaluate!

Lack of accountability simply paves the way to mediocrity.

Now that we have an understanding of the importance of holding each student accountable for their learning and growing, let's move on to reinforcement (feedback). While many faculty feel uncomfortable delivering negative feedback, others believe this is the only way to educate nursing students. As we review **reinforcement (feedback),** we are going to ask you to refocus your camera lens and look at feedback as focusing on self-awareness.

The three types of reinforcement (feedback) are motivational, informational, and developmental.

Nonperformance or weak students must be confronted, but you need to do it in a way that creates commitment rather than grudging compliance or outright resistance.

I had a powerful lesson to reinforce this factor. I can still remember working with a group of nursing students in my clinical area. I was only with this group for 2 weeks while the full time faculty member was attending a convention. The dean had asked me to help her out while I had a few weeks home in between consultations. I enjoyed working with the group. There were numerous challenges, however, that mandated I provide informational and developmental feedback . During the last clinical day, the group brought me a plaque that said, *"The best clinical days we've ever had."* I must admit, I was speechless. (That just does not happen very often! Just ask my husband.) I was so very touched and honored and very SURPRISED! Yet, I did not understand what made this clinical experience any different from the other days, so I asked. Their response, *"You actually gave us some positive feedback! We felt motivated! When we did have a challenge with a new procedure or a new assessment, you not only assisted us, but you talked us through the process after the skill so we understood the information. During that process, you gave us an opportunity to review what was supposed to happen, what actually happened, and what we would do differently next time. We actually learned as much from this process as we did from implementing the skill."* They went on to say, *"Typically we have only been given negative feedback and had felt that we would never be able to be a nurse. It was just too overwhelming. In fact we have asked our instructor to please tell us what she wants, and she would refer us to a 10 page evaluation. During the clinical prior to you working with us, we would just try to stay out of our instructor's sight so we would not get reprimanded! We decided to attempt to survive and just get by! One of our friends who is brilliant and loved nursing just withdrew because she felt so very incompetent every week. If only she could have heard just ONCE that she was doing something right."*

That was such a lesson and to tell you the truth I had no idea that I was making a difference! I just knew I loved them, loved nursing and loved the patients. I was so pleased to hear this because I did have a reputation for setting very high standards, but the students stretched and met the expectations. Does this have a familiar ring?

"EAR", Expectations, Accountability, Reinforcement, it works! That was the day I promised myself that I would continue to develop the habit of providing feedback to each student daily.

Of course, the challenge comes when the feedback is and cannot be positive. This is real! *All of us want to help students to become nurses, but there MUST be standards and expectations fulfilled to reach this outcome.* This group of clinical students taught me that negative feedback can also be energizing but in a different way. When somebody is told in a negative manner that he has fallen short of what was expected of him / her , there is a feeling of punishment. The result may renew the effort to perform better, but not always. Some students will run and hide from the instructor! Does this sound familiar? So what is our path to successful feedback?

We know that "no feedback" equates to extinction. This can be more punishing than negative feedback. It is the least motivating response one can make to any action. I hear colleagues say, *"I can't believe at the end of this clinical that the student is still not competent with medication administration."* I respond with, *"What kind of feedback did you give to the student?"* Their response, *"They need to continue practicing and have a better understanding of the process!"* If this is all the student is given, then it opens up the probability that poor performance is likely to be repeated or even grow worse. On the other hand, if you make no response to reinforce someone's good performance, even a minimal improvement, you will extinguish their motivation to improve.

If we want improvement, we have to reinforce improvement!

Why is this true? The reason is that once you get a pattern started, it takes only a small amount of reinforcement to keep it rolling. A habit is like a car; it is hard to start moving, but once it is rolling down the interstate, it only takes a little push on the gas pedal to keep it going. If you stop accelerating the gas pedal, the car will eventually stop. If you stop reinforcing desirable behavior altogether, that behavior will eventually stop.

When I have to deliver feedback regarding performance challenges (developmental), I have adapted "**ISSUE**" to assist with this process.

ISSUE	
I	Issue
S	Solutions
S	State options for improvement
U	Use reinforcement for positive responses
E	Exit

I will begin our discussion by stating the performance issue. I will make it a plain statement. For example, *"I have noticed that you are not implementing the 5 rights to medication administration consistently."* I make no judgmental statements, do not pass blame, and do not attempt to evaluate the problem. There is no reason for the student to become defensive. It is not negative or positive; it just is. Think of your statement as a mirror for the student to reflect and assist with self-awareness. If the information is stated clearly and indisputably, not loaded with blame, the student will be more aware of the behavior that needs changing. As we all know, many times it is not what we say but how we say it.

The second step is to elicit **solutions** without presenting questions that are historical in nature, that can be answered yes or no, and that begin with 'why' or 'who'. Think of **HOW** versus **WHO**! This acronym serves a double purpose. It shows us what not to say, but still reminds us to begin the interaction with **HOW**.

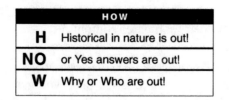

HOW	
H	Historical in nature is out!
NO	or Yes answers are out!
W	Why or Who are out!

We do not want excuses for the challenges; we want how to correct the challenge positively in the future. I use statements such as '**How can this be corrected?** or **What can we do to reverse this trend?**" These elicit positive statements regarding how the student can improve. If the student can articulate how the challenge can be corrected or a behavior improved, then the brainwork most likely has already been done. The clinical group that I discussed earlier indicated that this was an effective strategy to facilitate growth. They are novices! We must provide specific guidance.

The third step is to **state options**. I always think of this step as a brainstorming session. I do not evaluate their thoughts. Once the student has indicated several options for improving the clinical behavior, then I assist them with identifying which of the ideas could realistically be implemented. For example, with the above performance issue regarding medication administration several options for improvement may be as follows:

1. To review the 5 rights prior to clinical.

2. To make a concept map and carry it in my pocket to review in clinical.

3. To articulate this to my instructor prior to going into the room without being reminded.

4. Develop an image in my mind of this process.

5. Design a story in my mind regarding the consequences of not implementing the 5 rights to medication administration.

The fourth step is to **use reinforcement.** I reinforce any useful suggestions made.

For example, the next clinical day the student reviews the 5 rights with me and actually implements it successfully throughout the day. I provide him / her with positive reinforcement. If the student, however, continues to ignore this nursing activity, I ask again the **HOW** or **WHAT** questions outlined above. They will get it! *Remember, you learned to walk because your parents loved you and continuously reinforced you. They did not beat* *you up each time you fell!*

The fifth step is to **exit**. What I do here is to summarize everything we have discussed. I am getting the student's commitment to accomplish a specific task and obtain certain results. For example, I think we have agreed that for our patient's safety it is important to observe and implement the 5 rights of medication administration. We discussed several options to assist you in improving this behavior and that your best approach would be to review this with your instructor without being questioned, to carry a concept map in your pocket to jog your memory prior to this becoming a habit, and review consequences if a mistake is made. I end on a note that I believe in them and know they can make this happen. At this time, we decide on a date to revisit this activity.

Clinical Teaching and evaluation cannot be a hit and miss affair. It must be planned and coordinated to utilize the short period of time that we have to teach and the student has to learn. **As a clinical instructor you have the power to make a positive difference in the lives of everyone you touch!** The choice to select this path is open to you. I hope you choose to make a positive difference!

Chapter 10

PATHWAY TO TESTING: WHAT TO WRITE THE EXAM ITEMS ON

"Let the beauty we love be what we do,
There are hundreds of ways to kneel and kiss the ground"
Rumi

Many people think that all they have to do is to learn Bloom's Taxonomy and they will know how to write a test. How to write a test item is NOT the most important thing about the test. *The most important issue in test construction is WHAT TO WRITE THE ITEMS ON!* We have consulted with many programs where all faculty had PhD's and knew Bloom's like the back of their hand, but their graduates were making less than a 75% pass rate on the NCLEX-RN™ which is the minimum standard of safety.

How do we know what to write the items on? We use a BLUEPRINT. I don't know about you, but when I took an item writing course in graduate school, I promised myself to never use another blueprint. It was way too involved, had far too many threads, too many integrated pieces. It took me hours just to figure out what I should write the items about. Then why am I preaching BLUEPRINT? Because we need a minimum guide.

Many current faculty are using time as their blueprint. For example, "Mary, you had two hours of class; I need 20 items from you. John you had 3 hours of class, I need 30 items from you. Suzan, you had 1 hour of class I need 10 items from you. That makes a total of 60 items and that will be our test for next week." Time is one way to divvy out the number of items that need to be written, but it says nothing about what Mary, John and Suzan should write the items about.

I can hear you say, of course, they should write the items on their lecture or class presentation and you would be absolutely right IF they used the strategies laid out in Chapter 6 that discussed how to prioritize their class content. Go back and take a look at SAFETY.

SAFETY
System Specific Physical Assessment
Accuracy of orders and assignments to ancillary personnel (include room assignments)
Firsts – How to Prioritize (Which client to care for <u>first</u>, which light to answer <u>first</u>, which client to assess first, which piece of equipment that should be available <u>first</u>…)
Evaluate pharmacology (Drug/drug/food/herbs/dietary supplements/appropriateness of medication for this client, the 5 rights of medication administration.) How can the client live taking this medication for the rest of his life. What should his therapeutic blood level be? If it is too high what does the nurse do, too low?
Try infection control (as Yoda says, "Don't try, do")
Your assets, which means to write items on issues that will threaten your license. (Confidentiality, falls, lack of reporting nonfunctioning equipment or staff etc.)

Now, we have a BLUEPRINT. There are at least 10 concepts in the acronym SAFETY that can be used as a blueprint regarding what to write items about. These concepts all have priority in the current minimum standards as set by the NCSBN.

The NCSBN completes research every three years to update the minimum standards. For this reason, we, as nursing faculty, must take advantage of the new research to update the concepts in SAFETY, that will affect our priorities in teaching, clinical assignments, clinical evaluations and blueprint for our test items.

Some faculty have test banks that they have been using for years, not realizing that the standards change every three years. "Suddenly", they find that their students are not doing so well on NCLEX and they cannot understand why. All of us can learn from the book, *Who Moved My Cheese* written by Spencer Johnson M.D. It's the story about change. Little mice were fat and happy because their cheese was always in the same place. One day they went to eat and their cheese had been moved! "Suddenly" they were not doing well. Change takes place in the National Council of State Board Standards every three years. *We as nursing faculty cannot be in a position of using an old blueprint, old objectives, old content, old questions, or old ideas when we teach nursing. Nursing is too fluid and significant and we are way too smart for that.*

Chapter 11

PATHWAYS TO CONSTRUCTION OF CLINICAL REASONING EXAM ITEMS

"If you hear a voice within you saying,
You are not a painter, then by all means paint...
and that voice will be silenced "
Vincent Van Gogh

It is incredible how many nursing professors are using commercial test banks for their test items. It is incredible because many of the test banks that are published with text books are known to contain knowledge based items. This type of item allows the student to find the answer on a specific page in the text book. Educators that want to keep it real cannot stop item writing at this level of knowledge. In order to safely care for clients, learners of nursing have to utilize this knowledge to make a clinical decision regarding their actions. They utilize the knowledge to know which assessment to make next, analyze this assessment, plan their next action, implement their action and last, but not least, evaluate their action to see if it worked.

By now, you are saying, "The nursing process! Right on!" If the questions are not written regarding a client and the nurses' problem solving process, it probably is not a clinical reasoning item. *Our experience indicates that 85% of all items should be clinical reasoning items in order for the student or new graduate to be considered safe.* These items have a much higher difficulty level than knowledge based questions. Nursing uses a high level of intelligence to make clinical decisions. Our learners deserve to see and practice clinical reasoning items before they get to the NCLEX-RN™ . A clinical reasoning item is the kind of item that they have to think about. They may never find the answer to this type of question on a specific page in their text book. They will have had to synthesize many pages from many types of books to answer clinical reasoning questions.

Writing clinical reasoning items must start from DAY 1. Let me give you an example of the difference between a knowledge based item and a clinical reasoning item that can be utilized on the first test.

KNOWLEDGE
The normal body temperature is
1. 98.6
2. 101.6
3. 103.6
4. 106

Of course the answer is number 1. You said it in your lecture. The student has it backed up on their digital tape recorder. You can find it on a page in the text book. The student gets the answer correct, gets the point and is happy. This is definitely not a clinical reasoning item. There is no nursing process or any clinical reasoning involving a client in this type of item.

Take a look at the same concept written as a clinical reasoning item.

CLINICAL REASONING ITEM
The hospitalized client's temperature is 98.8. The nurse will now:
1. Sponge the client with a cool liquid.
2. Cover the client with a warm blanket.
3. Document the finding.
4. Notify the provider of the reading.

The answer, of course is number 3, but the student says, "Wait a minute. We discussed 98.6. We did not discuss 98.8. You cannot test anything that you did not teach!" Sound familiar? Here is an answer. "I really want to know if .2 of a point is enough to sponge the client with a cool liquid?" Students will think for a minute and then answer, "no". You tell them that their response is correct and ask them what they should do? Document it of course.

You may never be able to find 98.8 as a normal temperature on a specific page in the text book, but I hope you have discussed a range of normal in their class and discussed what to do if it is too high or too low.

This same type of item can be used with normal ranges of just about everything. It is not enough to know the normal ranges, the learner must know what to do when the client's range is outside of normal regardless of whether it is blood pressure, hemoglobin, BUN, blood glucose and any other objective approach. They have to know this from the first day that they learn the content. We have to begin our teaching using clinical reasoning as the core for learning.

We really want you to know what a knowledge based item looks like. We have seen hundreds of them while completing analysis of teacher made items during faculty development workshops. These items are written in the smallest associate degree program and in the largest most prestigious baccalaureate programs.

KNOWLEDGE BASED ITEMS
What were the major concerns of the ANA during the 1960's?
What were the objectives of the NLN during the 1970's
What was the Goldmark Report?
What war did Florence Nightingale fight in?
What part of the personality does the person with anti-social behaviors exhibit?
How many arteries and how many veins are in an umbilical cord?
The chief function of the ovaries is...
All of the following drugs are nitrates except...
All of the following drugs are ace inhibitors except...
All of the following drugs are beta blockers except...
All of the following drugs are insulin preparations except...
What part of One Minute Manager makes this a best seller?
Which of Lewen's management theories best demonstrates the nursing process?
The type of tumor classification that can be provided from a needle biopsy is?
During the Renaissance, the frequency of trade increased. Which disease did Not rise along with the trade?
Which drug should the doctor prescribe for these symptoms?
What should the nurse suspect that the doctor will use for treatment?
What is this client's medical diagnosis?
As Yul Brenner in the King and I said, "Etc, etc, etc."

We could go on for pages, probably another whole book. Do you see ANY clinical reasoning in any of these questions? Is there any patient involved? Is knowing any of these facts going to be a life and death situation or make the client safe? NO! Then WHY are we continuing to write this type of low intellect question?

I hear your brain thinking. Some of these questions were history questions. Are we not supposed to be teaching or testing history? Of course, we are supposed to be teaching history. How can we know where we're going if we don't know where we've been? At least bring some relevance into the history lessons. What difference does it make that Florence Nightingale fought in the Crimean War? The significant factor is that Florence believed that, cleanliness is next to Godliness. How can we fit this into our world of nosocomial infections? What significance did the historical reports have to do with where we find ourselves in nursing today?

Nursing students are adult learners. They want relevance or they only remember your history fact long enough to take the test. *Give them relevance.*

We can find the following type of question in virtually every college of nursing in the United States.

The blood gases are the following: the pH is x, the pCO2 is x, the HCO3 is x. The client is in:
A.   metabolic acidosis
B.   respiratory acidosis
C.   metabolic alkalosis
D.   respiratory alkalosis

It's as if someone is going to stand at the foot of the patient's bed and exclaim, "ah, respiratory acidosis"!

Let's turn this familiar question into one that is useful as a clinical reasoning item.

The client's pH is x, PCO2 is x, PCO3 is x. What should the nurses' next action be?
A.   Administer oxygen
B.   Place a paper sack over the clients mouth and nose
C.   Suction the client
D.   Put in an emergency call to the chief provider.

This question calls for clinical reasoning. The nurse takes the information and does something with it to make the client safe. There is a client involved. The nursing process is involved and this is a good question.

Many items ask questions about diseases or content questions. The nurse has to know more than just the information on the disease. Does this mean that we should not teach diseases? No, but it does mean that we can take a concept such as hyper or hypoglycemia and teach all of the diseases that cause these problems. Connect the issues for the learner and then ask them which assessment to make next, which laboratory test to analyze, which plan has priority, which implementation to begin first, or how to know that their nursing actions have worked.

We find many "Gotcha" type questions on faculty-made exams. Here is a prime example.

What kind of native American was in the video film that you were assigned?

1. A 28 year old Navajo
2. A 17 year old Creek
3. A 20 year old Sioux
4. A 15 year old Choctaw

This question came from a very prestigious university where the faculty needed time out of class. They assigned the students a video to watch on their own time and then wrote a question to "get them" if they did not see the video. There is actually nothing wrong with utilizing videos as learning experiences. We all know that a picture is worth a thousand words. The point here is to ask a question that is relevant to some nursing concept. Surely, there was a reason for the need to watch this important video. I seriously doubt that it was to determine which type of Native American starred in the film. Perhaps it was a sensitive cultural issue that the learner needed to grasp. Whatever it was, write the question on the issue.

There are more simple ways to construct good test items. For easier item construction we have put together a list of *Bottom-line questions*. The instructor can utilize these to be the "bottom lines" of questions that they need to write on their content. We include several of them for you to use. Note that we have listed them according to the nursing process so that you can vary your items. In other words, write some questions on assessment, some on implementation, etc.

BOTTOM LINE QUESTIONS

ASSESSMENT

Which vital sign should be (documented, followed up, discussed with other team members)?

Which client should be assessed first?

Which assessment would be a priority for this client (increased BP, decreased blood sugar, SOB, fluid draining from ears, vaginal bleeding, etc.)?

Which assessment best determines hydration status in this client?

ANALYSIS

Before this drug is administered the nurse should (check therapeutic blood level, check apical pulse, check allergies, etc.)

The most appropriate staff person to be assigned to this client is

Which finding would interfere with the effective functioning of (tubes, catheters, arterial lines, ventilators, infusion pumps, IVs, oxygen administration, restraints, etc.)

The RN, LPN, CNS should be assigned to care for which client?

PLAN

Thirty minutes prior to or after this procedure the nurse should plan

Which plan would best (prevent aspiration, promote wound healing, protect the client from injury etc)?

Which group of foods, drugs, or over the counter supplements should the client plan to avoid?

Discharge instructions to this client should include…

IMPLEMENT

Which intervention would have the highest priority (which the 2nd, 3rd, and 4th priority)?

From protocol choose the best intervention for the client with (bradycardia, tachycardia, non-captured pacemaker, respiratory arrest, cardiac arrest, choking etc.)

Which techniques demonstrate safe protocol when (discontinuing a chest tube, IV, decreasing pain, increasing vascular perfusion, protecting the client from self injury, caring for a client on a ventilator etc.)

What is your best response?

EVALUATION

Which evaluation would indicate a therapeutic response to this (drug, infection, procedure, hydration, alternative therapy)?

Which documentation would be most appropriate?

Which client concern is the most important?

Which measurement is most appropriate concerning (NG drainage, Lab results, intake and output records, vital signs etc)?

Do you see how these can be utilized to make your item writing easier? Actually, this page may be worth the whole price that you paid for this book.

We have clients that have used our bottom line questions for years to construct their items more quickly and simply. Just remember, every three years when the standards change and the cheese moves, these should be revised.

One key to writing excellent questions that evaluate thinking is to use a "**PATH**". This will simplify the "**PATH**" to writing these questions.

PATH	
P	Plausible distracters
A	Application
T	Thinking is multilogical
H	Has a focus on NCLEX-RN™ Activities (SAFETY)

Let's review this acronym in order to facilitate your success in writing questions that evaluate thinking.

Plausible distracters: Distracters should represent interventions or options (i.e., assessments, plans, etc.) that are appropriate for the client and /or condition described in the stem of the question. The reader must discriminate from among these similar interventions (options) in order to determine what should be done first or what has the highest priority. Students must learn that in a clinical situation the one best answer that typically appears in the text book may not be available when a clinical decision must be made. This can be challenging for the novice who is looking for only one right answer. This process of requiring high levels of discrimination to answer questions assists students with practice in making clinical decisions.

Application: The majority of questions are written at the application or a higher cognitive level *(Bloom's Cognitive Levels)*. The majority of test items are not written to evaluate knowledge or comprehension, but are prepared to evaluate clinical decision making.

Thinking is multilogical: Multilogical thinking is defined by Paul (1993) as: *"Thinking that sympathetically enters, considers, and reasons within multiple points of view."* The bottom line is that the reader is able to view problems from different perspectives. The questions require an understanding of both application and knowledge of a minimum of two concepts to answer successfully.

Has a focus on NCLEX-RN™ Activities (SAFETY): These bottom line questions will assist you with this process. Refer to above information.

Chapter 12

PATHWAY TO CURRICULUM PLANNING, AGENCY APPROVAL AND ACCREDITATION

"Simplify, Simplify."
Henry David Thoreau

By now, you are probably asking yourself, "Why was this not the first chapter? After all, you have to have at least agency approval and a curriculum plan before you have a college of nursing." Accreditation, of course, is a voluntary quest for cream of the crop status.

The reason this is not the first chapter is that it is not the most important. *The most important issue in any college of nursing is the actual teaching itself.* Teaching in the classroom and clinical teaching are paramount in the preparation of safe nurse clinical practitioners. We have witnessed a variation of curriculum plans that range from having been copied from the internet, to being developed by the entire faculty, to the brain child of a highly paid consultant. We have watched them all work or not. It's not what is in that plan. *It is what goes on between the teacher and the student.* That's why this chapter is late in the book. When we know what will go on in the classroom from developing relationships, to setting priorities, to providing competent and safe nursing care, we will have no problem planning the curriculum.

The biggest issue may be that someone has written a curriculum plan before you get there. It's ok. The real problem is how to revise it in the least offensive way to get it to reflect the concepts and values that have been laid out in this book. Most universities allow faculty to revise objectives without going through a time consuming curriculum committee. You need to try to stay out of those curriculum committee meetings. They will kill you in there. You don't have to change the course numbers or even the course names to accomplish great teaching. Do not use the curriculum plan as an excuse.

Great teaching is an easy accomplishment to write about for agency approval and accreditation. These agencies want the college of nursing to be successful. As long as the college can prove that it has a good plan, (even if it came off the internet), great teaching, satisfied students, good pass rates on the minimal standard test, the NCLEX, content graduates and pleased agencies that hire their products then, the approval and accrediting agencies will be assured.

It is our hope that universities will give more recognition and higher salaries to great teachers. It is the teacher's responsibility to document this "great teaching" so that they can document a reason for receiving promotion and tenure. We, as nursing faculty, have to show the university that great teaching is valuable. Sometimes they don't get it and teaching faculty are not rewarded as highly as the researchers or the community service faculty. It is up to us to make our case.

Accreditation can be a nightmare for a faculty that has to prepare a "self study" on top of everything else that they are doing. Remember, tell them what you are doing to meet their criteria and prove to them that you are doing this. That's the path to easy accreditation.

Chapter 13

PATHWAY TO LIFELONG LEARNING

"So great a power is there of the soul upon the body, that whichever way the soul imagines and dreams, thither doth it lead the body"
Agrippa, 1510

Isn't it ironic that the chapter on lifelong learning turns out to be chapter 13? Especially since we know that there is absolutely no bad luck in continuing to update ourselves. The important thing seems to be that we update ourselves. The concepts in this book have included relationships, collaboration, ownership, empowerment, and engagement among many others. These are not just concepts for teaching nursing. These are concepts for living.

In the past we have presented workshops on "Beyond Survival". We felt like it was our path to enlighten others that we are in this life to thrive not just to survive. We are in it because there is an abundance of joy and love in whatever we choose, if we choose to see it in this way. The quote on our first page reads, "We are what we think. All that we are arises from our thoughts. With our thoughts we make the world". We certainly make our own world. When we quit reading, listening or talking about relationships or nursing safety, or any of the other concepts in this book, that is when we quit having the thoughts that make our world full of joy and wealth. *Pathways to teaching nursing are pathways to abundance rather than scarcity.*

Read and listen about where the cheese is moving to next. Read and listen to information on behaviors that enhance and empower. Read and attend continuing education courses on the latest concepts that make nursing safe. Read and listen to the latest techniques of teaching and technology. Then, put all of these facts into perspective and dwell on the importance of every single one of them. Students do not learn from facts alone. Utilize yourself as a means to facilitate their learning. This will make lifelong learning imperative.

Of course, it takes courage to be a lifelong learner. Backing away from challenges and new situations often ends up blunting learning and blocking us from discovering new ways to make a difference. As Anais Nin put it, *"Life shrinks or expands in proportion to one's courage."* It is heartening to realize that while human beings may crave comfort, rituals, and routine, we truly nourish the soul's growth primarily through what is difficult and challenging. As Darwin saw it, *"It's not the strongest of the species that survives, nor the most intelligent, but those who are most responsive to change."*

After all, transformation is a lifelong experience that will be forever a part of who you are, so enjoy this path of "lifelong learning" all along your journey. We hope you will enjoy your path as much as we have enjoyed and continue to enjoy ours! Thank you for sharing this part of your path with us!

Afterword

UNITING RESEARCH AND PRACTICE

Melissa J. Geist, PhD, RN

The goal of research in education is to systematically investigate new and innovative ways to teach in order to influence how students learn. It is a complex fusion of theory and practice. The authors of *Pathways* have compiled a powerful guide to teaching student nurses based on 45 years of experience working with nurses at all levels and in all settings. Not surprisingly, the ideas presented in this book are also reflected by current research in the science of learning. *Pathways* is the ideal bond between practical expertise and learning theory.

The National Research Council (NRC) (2000) published *How People Learn: Brain, Mind, Experience and School*, a synthesis of research in cognitive development and the learning sciences. The book describes effective learning environments as being Learner-centered, Knowledge-centered, Assessment-centered, and Community-centered. Just as the authors of *Pathways* stress the importance of renewal of an entire nursing program, these components of effective learning environments must be considered as an inseparable unit. It is worth taking a closer look at how the strategies presented in this book align with the *How People Learn* framework.

Learner-Centered Environments

Learner-centered environments take into account the fact that learners do not enter our classrooms as "blank slates." Students, and nursing students to an even greater degree, come with skills, knowledge and beliefs shaped from other aspects of their lives. "Teachers who are learner centered recognize the importance of building on the conceptual and cultural knowledge that students bring with them to the classroom" (NRC, 2000, p. 134). The science education literature refers to "diagnostic teaching"; meaning the teacher is constantly gathering information about each student's perspective by observing, questioning, and engaging the student in conversation (Geist, 2004; Lemke, 1990; Warren & Rosebery, 1996).

Rayfield and Manning tap into this research by urging nursing professors to elicit and value student contributions through "shared expectations, communications and ownership". One of the most valuable recommendations can be found in the 'E' of the RESPECT acronym, "we should ask where they are and what they need." This statement is the essence of a learner-centered environment; continuous monitoring of the cognitive and emotional state of each student.

Knowledge-Centered Environments

A strictly learner-centered environment would obviously not ensure that our students become safe, effective, and professional nurses. They must have an extensive information base, which begins with prior knowledge that is progressively formalized. As the formalization of knowledge proceeds, students should learn how to use the information in a variety of contexts (Schwartz, Lin, Brophy, & Bransford, 1999). For example, it is no longer appropriate to isolate and teach pharmacology in a single pharmacology course. Students must be able to think about medication administration across patient care settings. If we teach pharmacology in a single context, we should not be surprised that students can only apply the knowledge in that context. "With multiple contexts, students are more likely to abstract the relevant features of concepts and develop a more flexible representation of knowledge" (NRC, 2000, p.78). *Pathways* reiterates the necessity of identifying priority concepts and then revisiting these concepts with an increasing degree of complexity throughout the entire nursing program. With this approach student nurses learn the most relevant content as they apply knowledge in a variety of circumstances.

Assessment-Centered Environments

Assessment centered environments are designed with several opportunities to provide feedback and to allow students to rethink and revise. These classrooms are also characterized by careful alignment of assessments with the stated objectives of the unit. Both formative and summative assessments should be included to properly track students' learning. Formative assessments are generally administered in the classroom and serve as sources of feedback to make students' thinking visible. Summative assessments are the more traditional tests to measure learning at the end of a unit. The authors provide excellent techniques for aligning nursing goals with assessments, and for measuring students' learning.

One area of nursing education in immediate need of improvement is clinical evaluation. The typical nursing program requires students to write lengthy, time-consuming care plans on their assigned patient and this care plan provides the basis for the clinical grade. It is certainly no secret that most students copy these care plans from books, therefore we are assessing what students can copy, not what they can do. The authors suggest that educators need to "TRACK" students' progress starting with the development of basic technical skills moving toward the development of clinical reasoning to manage multiple complex client cases.

Community-Centered Environments

Although all four components of effective learning environments recommended by the NRC (2000) are absolutely necessary, the community-centered aspect is at the heart of *Pathways*. Community-centered environments facilitate collaboration and relationship building in the interest of furthering student learning. Again and again Rayfield and Manning stress the importance of creating an atmosphere of mutual respect between the instructor and the students, but they do not stop at this surface level. The community goes beyond the classroom; it includes the university, the clinical agencies, even the larger locale in which the school of nursing is situated. Taking students to the local shopping mall to conduct blood pressure screenings not only motivates the students, it builds valuable relationships between the school and the greater community. With this model nursing students identify with becoming a valuable health care provider in the first weeks of school. They begin their journey toward becoming a professional nurse.

Change is taking place in nursing education. It is no longer appropriate or effective to adhere to the "blank slate" view of instruction. Students are not empty vessels waiting to be filled with information; they are complex individuals with developed identities and beliefs. Current research in cognitive development and the science of learning has shown that genuine learning takes place when instruction is learner, knowledge, assessment and community centered. This model has been implemented in biomedical engineering programs at some of the most prestigious universities in the country with incredible results (Brophy, 2003). Sylvia Rayfield and Loretta Manning have created a guide for nurse educators to do the same. They have provided a pathway to a new and exciting era in nurse education.